The Love Knot

Ties That Bind
Cancer Partners

"The world of cancer and loved ones affects every relationship, and can leave permanent devastation. As the proud daughter to one of America's legends, Michael Landon, I urge any participant in cancer to read this book as a vital guidebook to live deliberately so that cancer partnership can be used with grace, comfort, and knowledge. Knowledge is empowerment and empowerment is wisdom . . . this is our most powerful tool to deal with the blinding effects of cancer that makes us feel out of control and hopeless. To walk into a cancer situation blind and ignorant is like the blind leading the blind . . . you fall into a dark pit. This book serves wisdom forming *ideas* of the cancer partnership and what *it feels* to share the cancer with all relationships using deliberate guidance allowing each participant in cancer to **know purposeful living, offering greater meaning to the disease.** Without the deliberate guidance Robert Ross offers we face devastation and painful memories. With his guidance we discover the true love knot tying purpose to our hearts. I wish I had read this book when my Dad faced his $2\frac{1}{2}$ month fight with cancer, leaving an agony of loss that goes beyond the pages."

—Cheryl Landon,
author, radio producer and hostess,
professional inspirational seminar speaker,
teacher, and mother

World Headquarters
Jones and Bartlett Publishers
40 Tall Pine Drive
Sudbury, MA 01776
978-443-5000
info@jbpub.com
www.jbpub.com

Jones and Bartlett Publishers Canada
2406 Nikanna Road
Mississauga, Ontario
CANADA L5C 2W6

Jones and Bartlett Publishers International
Barb House, Barb Mews
London W6 7PA
UK

PRODUCTION CREDITS
ACQUISITIONS EDITOR: Penny Glynn
PRODUCTION EDITOR: Linda S. DeBruyn
EDITORIAL/PRODUCTION ASSISTANT: Christine Tridente
MANUFACTURING DIRECTOR: Therese Bräuer
TYPESETTING AND TEXT DESIGN: Peter G. Schiller
PRINTING AND BINDING: Malloy Lithographing, Inc.
COVER DESIGN: Anne Spencer

Library of Congress Cataloging-in-Publication Data
Ross, Robert N., 1941–
    The love knot : ties that bind cancer partners / Robert N. Ross.
      p. cm.
    ISBN 0-7637-1412-7 (pbk. : alk. paper)
      1. Cancer--patients--Family relationships. 2.
Cancer--Psychological aspects. I. Title.

    RC254.5 .R67 2001
    362.1'96994--dc21

                                                    00-055822

Printed in the United States of America
04 03 02 01 00   10 9 8 7 6 5 4 3 2 1

The Love Knot

Ties That Bind
Cancer Partners

Robert N. Ross

JONES AND BARTLETT PUBLISHERS

Sudbury, Massachusetts

BOSTON   TORONTO   LONDON   SINGAPORE

Contents

Preface

My wife Trudee and I lived for almost three years with a rare form of cancer known as leiomyosarcoma. She was the one who had the cancer, but in every other way we both were stricken by the disease. Even though she eventually died, I would say that together we got through this challenging time with considerable grace. Trudee, I think, would say the same.

Partners of people with cancer face a bitterly sweet conflict: We are beset by sharp pangs of anguish, but if we didn't also feel love, we wouldn't feel that anguish. That powerful interweaving of many contradictory strands—love, fear, hope, anguish, expectation, anger, shared history, and lost future—is what I call the love knot. In the cancer life, that knot is both the sweet bond that ties two people together in trust and love, and the tight constrictor knot that binds two people in bitterness and fear.

What is surprising about what Trudee and I went through is that so much of our cancer experience was positive. If our experience had been the unmitigated disaster that we all expect cancer to be, there would have been no point in writing this book. I felt a strong desire to write this book precisely because our experience was unexpected.

Our life together in the cancer world would certainly have been less rewarding if not for Trudee's gallantry. She loved her life, which cancer only made more precious. She told me more than once that I was her reason for living, that she would not have had the strength to endure her private cancer pains without me. I still believe her. Her struggle to maintain her life in the face of ultimate disaster made my own life more precious, too.

We who play the role of cancer partner have very few models, as each person's cancer experience is different. I have written this book in the hope that some portion of Trudee's and my experience might live beyond us, not to serve as a model, but to help other people in the cancer world live their own versions of this powerful, overwhelmingly human drama.

Foreword

The role of Cancer Partner is unlike any other role that a person will play in the course of a lifetime, and it is one for which—until now—there has been little guidance or support. The person diagnosed with cancer faces challenges and experiences that the cancer partner cannot even begin to comprehend; however, the cancer partner also faces unique challenges. Only a cancer partner knows what it feels like to reassure his wife that she is beautiful even as her hair falls out; or to care for her husband while he grows weaker, taking care not to damage his sense of strength and independence.

The cancer partner role is an essential one in the life of the cancer patient. Robert Ross's very personal, yet universal, description of the ups and downs of being a cancer partner will help many people who are struggling daily with their own experiences with cancer while caring for their loved ones. Whether new or a veteran to the role, cancer partners in all stages of the experience will be able to relate to Ross's story of himself and his wife Trudie, and identify with their journey through the cancer world. Although the journey is different for each couple, the goals of making that journey well may be similar for all couples: cherish the time together; hold on to each other; make memories . . . and then treasure and honor those memories when they are all that remain.

The Love Knot: Ties that Bind Cancer Partners is Robert Ross's gift to those who live with the fear, the pain, the uncertainty, and possible loss of the person they love most in the world.

Pamela Willsey, LICSW
Program Director
Wellness Community—Greater Boston

Partners in the Cancer World

Partnership at will: One designed to continue for no fixed period of time, but only during the pleasure of the parties, and which may be dissolved by any partner without previous notice.

— ***Black's Law Dictionary***

Many books have been written on how to be a cancer survivor, on how to make the necessary accommodations to cancer without being defeated by it, on how not to act the victim. Not surprisingly, these books have been written primarily for the person who actually has cancer. But the intrusion of a life-threatening illness like cancer touches a circle of people far beyond the person who has cancer. For everyone who has been brushed—even if only lightly—by the "Big Crab," all previous time seems impossibly innocent. Yet although the partner's role is equally difficult to play well, no book about living with cancer is devoted primarily to the partner's side of the story.

It may seem self-indulgent to pay so much attention to the person who doesn't have cancer. In the best of worlds, both players in a crisis support each other equally. But the reality of living with cancer is that the person who is undergoing chemotherapy, who is in pain, or who is exhausted and frightened may not be able to support the partner in dealing with the other upsets of life in the cancer world. And who could find fault? The person with cancer is fighting for life. Cancer partners struggle with dreadful issues, too, but not literally for their own survival.

I have had the role of cancer partner thrust upon me, and I have talked with many other people who have likewise played that role. My

1

own experience and my conversations with fellow cancer partners have taught me much about this terrible and wonderful role. No other experience I can think of captures so perfectly the basic truth that life is an amalgam of pain and pleasure. Hope can hurt, and miraculously, even pain can have a life-affirming, positive side. Being a cancer partner teaches us the mixture of good and evil in the human state. It is no exaggeration to say that the experience gives us an opportunity to be the best a human being can be.

In our own little cancer world, the one inhabited by my wife Trudee and me, the cancer was *our* problem. Neither of us could escape it. We faced it together. When Trudee had a doctor's appointment, we both went. When she had her regular CT scans, we both sweated and fidgeted until the doctors told us the results. When Trudee had her MRIs, she was the one who squeezed into the machine's narrow tube, but I sat alongside while the machine clunked and whined. We gave each other the thumbs-up sign when the MRI platform finally slid her back out of the tube. If I could have taken half the chemotherapies for her, I would have.

The cancer accompanied us wherever we went, all the time. Sometimes it came as an unwanted intruder, causing momentary alarm, as when I hugged Trudee too tightly or somehow in the wrong way, and the mass she called her "evil twin" let us know it. Sometimes it came as a threatening sign, seen on the horizon of our lives, as when we first realized that her swelling was becoming outwardly visible without the aid of electronic imaging equipment.

Nothing we could do would bribe or trick the intruder into leaving us alone. We couldn't scare it away. We couldn't ignore it. Treatment to blast it away might help, but it might not. Actually, we were told that it probably would *not*. Trudee had a rare kind of cancer that did not lend itself to treatment. No one used the word "incurable," but we knew that there would be no happy ending to this adventure. Our only hope of getting through this time together was to come to terms with Trudee's cancer and learn how to coexist with it. We would not let the cancer come between us. Trudee and I shared a somewhat warped sense of humor, a deep faith in each other, and a philosophy of life that included looking over the edge into the Abyss (always with a capital A). We had acknowledged the Abyss before cancer, but we had never had to deal with it. The arrival of cancer in our lives changed all that.

We had known people who had "gotten cancer," but we had no idea how that intrusion shifted their center of gravity, individually and as couples. Cancer seems different from other serious illnesses. Heart disease, diabetes, and arthritis all impose terrible burdens on both the people who have the illnesses and their partners. But those diagnoses don't carry the sinister connotations of cancer. There is still something special about cancer. It carries such malign magic that people hesitate even to say the word. Trudee and I didn't know if people ever recovered their balance after receiving a diagnosis of cancer. If they did, how?

Trudee and I would not permit the cancer—or more specifically, the fear of separation caused by the cancer—to defeat us by driving us apart prematurely. Instinctively, for I would not pretend that we had thought out how to make something of her cancer, we drew closer together. Trudee threw herself into treatment even though she knew that therapy would certainly be hard and might be futile. More than once, she told me that she was joining the battle with her cancer out of love for me. I took on as much of the cancer burden as I could. Except for some of the obvious things that only she could do, we did as much as we could together. Why? For want of a better word, I'll call it love.

Everyone knows or can imagine the difficulties of the cancer life: fear, pain, fatigue, nausea, loss. Only people who have actually been there can also recognize that the experience can have a positive side. I will not idealize the painful, difficult, frightening, confusing, unwanted, and menacing cancer experience that has touched all of us who have entered the cancer world. Much of life in the cancer world is ugly and painful. Nobody with cancer goes there voluntarily. We should not expect living with cancer (and dying, if that should happen) to be a beautiful experience. Cancer stinks. It is a rotten disease. Within that terrible frame, however, many surprising things happen. There were moments during our time in the cancer world when the life Trudee and I shared was so clear and so powerfully charged with meaning that it is hard not to call the experience good.

Dealing with cancer is not easy. But good and easy are not synonymous. What *is* good, if we choose to see it, is that the disaster of cancer forces us to extract some meaning from our struggle to live with it. "Nevermore" is the saddest word in the English language. Philosophy and religion have struggled with the problems of love and nothingness for millennia. Cancer gives us the concrete opportunity to do so every day. To survive cancer relatively intact—even if one of the partners eventually dies—depends on our willingness and ability to find meaning in the details of the daily life we have left. We may not always succeed, but the cancer presents us—the partner and the person with cancer—with a rare opportunity to live a deliberate life.

It seems almost inconceivable, in retrospect, that the experience of watching the cancer threat play itself out would *not* change our lives. It would take an almost inhuman effort to pass through the experience of living with cancer unchanged. More importantly, it would be a terrible waste to have gone through such an experience without being changed by it. Our willingness to allow the change and to recognize it is probably the only meaning we can attach to this otherwise arbitrary, capricious, and inexplicable turn of luck.

The Biggest Surprise

Most of the time, the person we love seems to be both close and infinitely removed. We may feel close to our partners and still have only the sketchiest idea of what it feels like to live inside their skin. We know only what we can see, and then what we can imagine. From the sketchy facts available to us—she likes to work in the garden, the texture of chicken gristle makes him gag, she can sing all the lyrics of "The Midnight Train to Georgia"—we can barely imagine what life feels like from the inside. Collecting more details won't solve the problem, and normally, there isn't much reason to dwell on those speculations. In the short term, we are happy to be surprised by things that seem out of character. The more we love our partners, the more we can be surprised. "Out of character" simply means that we don't know everything yet; surprise shows that we are still learning and that we care.

Sharing the cancer experience can reduce that infinite gulf that separates us. The gulf between the person with the cancer and the cancer partner is still a yawning infinity, but it suddenly becomes important to bridge that chasm. Very few of our experiences take place in that half-infinite distance on the bridge we build over the void. Each of us may be profoundly moved by *The Marriage of Figaro*, for example, or by a sunset over the water, or by someone's gesture of kindness. In each of these experiences, we can be moved but still not *require* that our partner also feel moved. Not many experiences absolutely *require* that they be shared if they are to work at all.

The best example of an experience that must be shared in this way is that of falling in love. What does it feel like to fall in love? It would be presumptuous of me to try to describe the feeling; each one of us thinks we invented it and hold the patent. And in a way, we do. Aside from the intense concentration on just the world of the couple in love, there is also the effort, from one side and the other, to move into that half-infinite space between the lovers. We wonder what will make that other person laugh, what she would find interesting, what might be valuable to him, what would make her feel good.

The best way to find answers to these important lover's questions is by experiment. Try something. See what happens. Take a chance. You have to risk making a fool of yourself if you are going to learn anything. You could play it safe, but that's an experiment of a sort, too, and could just as easily make a fool of you.

That deeply wonderful (in all senses of the word, from "incalculably good" to "full of wonder") experience of being in love can serve as a model for how to live together in the cancer world. Octavio Paz has described love as the bet we make on the freedom of "the Other." The love-bet is that the Other will select us and will maintain that selection as if it mattered, above all. As with every bet, circumstances (perhaps chance, fate, or distance) must threaten the loss of what we value. Without the risk, there is no bet and no triumph.

Without the possibility that the Other *might* go away, there is no love. The risk of the Other going away, in fact, is what adds weight to the great wager of love. If we are talking about love, the person on each side of the infinite gulf is working hard to build a bridge across it. In other words, falling in love (as opposed to the one-sided affair known as obsession) is a shared experience that depends on reciprocity for its very life.

The business of living together with cancer is transacted in that same strange land of half-infinite distance. Living in the cancer world—not just surviving or tolerating the rigors of that bizarre existence, but really living in that world—can be very much like living in the world of romantic love. Who would have thought it! First of all, the initial bet—the ante to get into the game at all—is that the Other might go away. Without the threat of change, suffering, and death, the world of cancer would be a walk in the park. In truth, however, the terror that motivates everything else in dealing with cancer is the terror of pain and, ultimately, of separation.

Like falling in love, living together with cancer depends for its very life on sharing the experience. Like falling in love, living with cancer gets us out of ourselves and into that half-infinite distance. Like falling in love, living with someone else's cancer forces us to imagine life from inside that other person. We learn what is valuable to the Other. And, as in falling in love, the only way to learn what we need to know is by experiment. The experiment may be more fun in the love world than in the cancer world, but the results of the experiment are far more important in the cancer world.

Unfortunately, the pressure of living with cancer can drive out any inclination to experiment. Too much of life is out of control to allow the kind of playfulness and curiosity that this kind of experiment requires. We are not accustomed to living there, and so we can encounter many unusual problems. But how you live together through the cancer has a great impact on how the survivor feels if the worst nightmare comes to pass. If you can look back on the experience and say that you did the best you could, that in some ways living with the cancer brought out the best in both of you, you can look back on that time with positive feelings as well as sadness. The sadness is real, and it won't go away. But some of the good can be carried along, too.

The stupid, brute fact of Trudee's cancer forced us to deal meaningfully with all the changes it imposed on us. She and I resisted making some of those changes, and we kept up our familiar old life for as long as we could. We went to France. We bought a sailboat. We renovated the bathrooms. We bought groceries. We saw our friends. We acted as if we had a future. Eventually, we yielded, bit by bit, to the greater force of the cancer in our lives. But we relinquished only the things we did, not the ways we thought and related to each other. Trudee had to stop working and devote her energies to therapy. I had to make my work conform to the necessities of the moment in Trudee's therapy. In a very real sense, we had to give up our happy conventional life and embrace a new life of our own devising. We had to test the adequacy of our familiar roles with each other and feel our way into new roles when necessary.

Role of the Cancer Partner

Being the cancer partner is more complicated, in some ways, than being the person who has cancer. Whether people with cancer see themselves as victims or as sick people or as fighters or as survivors, the roles they play are clearly spelled out. Their roles are defined by the healthcare system, by the requirements of treatment, by conventional (and, incidentally, often quite mistaken) societal notions of what it is like to have cancer, and by their own beliefs about cancer. Their roles are also defined by their acceptance or rejection of the "sick role." Their personal history and psychological makeup shape and refine the role as it is played out.

The roles of the partner, on the other hand, are not so clearly defined and are not so explicitly supported. The role of the cancer partner is invented and re-invented every day. A brand of Scotch used to advertise that people were mature enough to drink the product when they could deal with the domestic question, "Honey, do I look fat in this dress?" The cancer partner deals with questions like this all the time. "I look awful without any hair, don't I?" "Am I getting too thin?" "Does it bother you that we can't walk in the woods the way we used to?" "Aren't you getting tired of seeing all those medicine bottles on the dresser?" "Have you notice how tired I'm looking these days?" "Do you think you will marry again?" Behind these apparently simple questions lie the worlds within worlds that make up another person. In our answers, too, are our own nested hopes and fears. For the partner of the person with cancer, there is also a lot of guessing and trying to understand, on sometimes flimsy evidence, how the partner is feeling. On top of that, the person with the cancer may not know what he or she needs or wants or be able to ask others for it if the need is clear. Little wonder, then, that it is so difficult to know how to give support when it is needed and in a form that speaks to that need. Both sides of the loving partnership are making an immense effort to buttress the crumbling bridge that spans the gulf between them. Clarity—feeling *and* thinking—is one of the first victims. Yet the cancer partner has to invent a clear role in this strange new world. Meanwhile, the threat of being the sole survivor of their shared story, living on in a much-changed world, is always lurking around the corner of the cancer partner's awareness.

The partners may also want to protect each other so much that they may not tell each other exactly what they sense, feel, or know. As a result, the two may be on different tracks at different times. When this happens, it can be very difficult for the partners to respond to each other in ways that count. Partners of those with cancer have their own needs and separate lives that they are trying to maintain. The partners with cancer have other needs. The two may be so far removed and so demanding in their different ways that it can be very difficult for them to confront their common experience of cancer. People do not necessarily arrive at the major waypoints of understanding the cancer experience at the same time. This is one of the biggest struggles.

In the past, there was no real support system for cancer partners. Recently, however, organizations like the Wellness Community offer regular support groups for family members of people with cancer as well as for people they refer to as "participants." Even for this enlightened organization, earlier thinking was that family members would be too exhausted to seek help for themselves. Since resources for support are limited, they thought, the effectiveness of support programs would be greater if they were devoted exclusively to helping the person with cancer. "Supporting the family members who are supporting the person with cancer is an important part of the whole process of dealing with cancer," says Pamela Willse, Executive Director of the Wellness Community of Greater Boston. "Working with family members came almost as an afterthought. It comes as part of an effort to strengthen the role of the family. Now we are trying to get back to the notion of supporting the family in this time of crisis."

Why This Book

This is not a history of Trudee's illness or the story of my involvement in it. I am writing, as truthfully as I can, about what it is like to be the other person in cancer, to be the one who lives with the cancer but is not the person who has it.

Trudee and I did not invent cancer and sickness. We are not the first people to feel the pain of a coming separation. I leave it to the students of the human condition to puzzle out how it is that we all live with foreseeable death and act as if it will come as a surprise. Perhaps there is something special, as in the case of cancer, in knowing the name of that death. Naming it makes it real in a way that seems impossible without the name. I also leave to the students of the psyche to figure out why we think that we were somehow singled out for such misfortune. What we went through was in no way unique—actually, it must have been quite commonplace—but it felt unique.

I fell in love with a woman who became the central point of my existence until, fifteen years later, I watched her die, and even eased her way a little. The thought of what I myself (and we together) went through pains me. The thought that she is forever lost to me and to the world that knew her and might have known her pains me. The belief that she died because of some mindless accident in coding the proteins that regulated some of her body's growth pains me. The trick now is to put words, and perhaps, therefore, meaning, to that hurt, inadequate as those words might be to the task.

The partner has an equal interest in the outcome and in the day-to-day events of life in the cancer world. But, as with any good partnership, although the two roles have a good deal in common, they also differ in important ways. Calibrating that distance between the partners so that it is close enough to be mutually satisfying but not so close that the boundaries disappear between the two partners is one of the difficult feats of dealing with cancer. Too close, and you both lose your autonomy. Too distant, and you lose intimacy. Done right, it comes as close as we can come to defeating death itself. Writing this book from the point of view of the partner who does not have the cancer is an effort to map that proper distance.

The practical necessities of dealing with cancer naturally create extraordinary stresses. As a result, many cancer partners say that they have serious regrets about how they performed their role. The sense of impotence can be overwhelming as the partner feels less and less able to do anything that might affect the course of the disease or the loved one's comfort. In some couples, the bonds strengthen, and they experience a renewed sense of mutual commitment. In other couples, however, the stresses of dealing with the illness increase the distance between them. Both men and women are forced to take on new roles in the household: Couples may not have a strict division of roles, but they may be forced by the incapacity of one of the members to take more than the usual share of the once-common burden. This shifting in conventional and well-understood roles may strain the relationship.

This book is about something other than how a man who may not have spent much time grocery shopping now must take over the family shopping, or how a woman who may not have dealt with taking the car to the mechanic must now negotiate a brake job. This book is about what happens when the two people in this intimate partnership must shift roles in the most unexpected and unwanted ways. When cancer comes into the couple's life, entire new roles must be invented. The person with the cancer must learn the intricacies of the sick role. The partner must invent on the spot the whole range of supporting roles.

Meanwhile, the person with cancer usually has little idea of what the other partner is going through. The partner may try to protect the other from the worst fears. While this is a natural and in some ways a helpful strategy, albeit an unconscious one, the slightest change in how the two partners relate to each other disrupts the delicate balance of trust. It leaves the person with cancer at a definite disadvantage, knowing that the partner is feeling pain, knowing that the pain is directly related to the cancer, and feeling that to raise the issue would be to involve the partner in a discussion of the very topics that the partner is trying to protect the other from.

There is no single formula for dealing with what cancer partners go through. This book is about how cancer partners deal with the uncertainty cancer brings, and how these partners help the person with cancer deal with the uncertainty. This book is about how to live within what seems to be a drastically foreshortened horizon of certainty. I hope this book is relatively free of prescriptive advice. I would not presume to tell you how to run your lives, with cancer or without. Every partnership experiences the cancer story from its own vantagepoint. In that regard, the number of different cancer stories is very large. Nevertheless, I am a veteran of the cancer world. Having lived through all phases of the cancer partnership, I can say the following with certainty:

1. Cancer is like life, only more so.
2. It need not all be bad.
3. Living the cancer partner's role takes great imagination.
4. If you do it well, the payoff is great.

The Defining Moment

Here the boundaries meet
And all contradictions exist side by side.
—*Fedor Mikhailovich Dostoevski,*
The Brothers Karamazov

I t's odd; you would think that a boundary as important as that between the old world and the cancer world would be clearly marked. The actual border is unforgettable; but the approaches to the cancer world are often so unremarkable that we barely notice when we have started our progress to the other side. Anyone who has entered the cancer world talks about that border crossing as one of the great divides in life. It is a line we cross only once, from innocence to cancer. Once that boundary is crossed, our lives are changed forever. If we come back across that border, we return as different people.

People who have been spared this experience cannot fully comprehend it. And people who have lived through such border crossings are often reluctant to talk about them with people who haven't, partly because they would rather leave their own painful memories undisturbed, but also because they realize how much must be explained to the uninitiated in order to give them an inkling of what they are talking about. Like people who have lived through battles, only people who have lived in the cancer world can understand that acts of gentleness and generosity in the trenches only *seem* to be anomalies. Who, then, are the fortunate ones? Those who lived through the horrors and have gained a stronger and deeper sense of humanity, or those who never saw them at all?

When discussing their border crossings, many cancer partners tell how an apparently trivial event turned out to be the moment that changed their lives. They describe their efforts to keep that event anchored in the familiar and recognizable world, despite what retrospect shows to be their inexorable progress toward the borderline between the old familiar world and the cancer world. The cancer partner often tags along good-naturedly, but in a careless way, on the paths that lead to the border. Generally, there is something "a little funny" that ought to be examined more closely, but nothing *really* to worry about. Rarely is the approach to the border marked by warning signs.

Then comes the border crossing itself. Suddenly, innocents that we are, we find ourselves surprised by the reality of our situation. We make one more turn, and then directly ahead we see the checkpoint. We approach the border bravely, still clutching at normalcy. Like raw immigrants arriving in a new land, we enter the cancer world carrying the few bags that contain our meager belongings. The bags hold what we imagine to be the necessities of daily living in the new world. Greenhorns like us believe that we will need only what had been necessary in that past life. But too soon it becomes obvious that we are entering a baffling new world. Still, in order to shore up our increasingly shaky sense of normalcy, we struggle to keep all our baggage with us, both the useful and the useless. It might be easier to leave the bags behind a rock near the border and to come back for them later when we are not so burdened, but carrying them is also comforting. We think that they are all we have, and the weight itself reminds us of something familiar.

People who visit unfamiliar places may be either travelers or tourists. Tourists seek out what is known and comfortable in the strange lands and return home with their sense of the familiar reconfirmed. Travelers, whether they want to or not, confront the particular and the personal in the strange lands they visit. The particular is always at least a little unfamiliar. Comfortable beauties of the new world may open up to travelers, but only after spending time there. In the first confusion of dislocation at the border, people hang on like displaced persons in wartime. They are waiting. They are not where their lives are. They have been alienated—but even that is not clear to them. They haven't yet been shocked into catching up with their new lives.

The new wayfarers in the cancer world sit in a crude inn not far from the border they just crossed. It is early evening and they are resting for the first time since having made the initial leg of their journey. They know nothing of what lies ahead, but they fear it. Their fear smolders like the damp logs in the large stone fireplace at the end of the common room they huddle in, and fills the room with the same kind of heavy smoke. The travelers feel cold. They feel cut off from what had been their lives. They are dazed by the turmoil of their recent days. They are tired, but too worked up to take rest. Some sit rigid, stolid, and silent. Others talk too loudly with an enforced jollity that seems oddly out of place in the dank and joyless inn.

We are a group none of us chose to join. Yesterday we knew nothing of each other. Today we are intimates. Our anxieties hold us together. Almost despite ourselves, we realize how much we have in common. Uneasily, haltingly because we don't know each other very well, a few of us begin to tell each other the stories of how we made our way to the border. The stories are like fragments of dreams. There is little of the larger contexts that once were our lives. As in a nightmare, the few facts are everything.

The First Traveler's Tale: Dorothy

A friend of mine was telling me that both her mother and her sister had a rare and aggressive form of brain tumor called glioblastoma. First her mother developed the cancer, then her sister developed the same thing. Her sister died in six weeks. I listened and gave what support I could as my friend told me that she was completely exhausted by her ordeal of caring for both her mother and her sister. We talked for a few hours over coffee.

When I got home, my husband was sitting on the porch—just sitting, which I thought was a little odd. I sat down in the chair facing him and started telling him my friend's sad story. We were face to face on the porch, our knees occasionally touching. As we talked, I felt so lucky to have him and to have the life we had. After I finished telling him my friend's story, I expected him to do what he had done so many times in the past: take my hand and say one of those wise and warm and supportive things that rarely failed to make me feel better. Instead, he said to me, "You know, it's a funny thing. I've had this headache all week." My husband had been working very hard at the time, so at first the doctors were sure that his headache was related to stress. They recommended relaxation exercises. When the exercises didn't help, we went back to the doctor. They did some tests and finally had a diagnosis: it was glioblastoma.

The Second Traveler's Tale: Cindy

After every cold, it was normal for my husband to have a cough that lingered for a few weeks, so we didn't think anything of it when he kept coughing for more than a month. We just thought that he had caught some especially tenacious kind of cold. "It will go away," we told each other. When his cough lasted for several months, we started to think that this cold might be different. "Why should I struggle with this cough when modern medicines can get rid of it in a week or so?" he said to me. I'll never forget that day. He went to the doctor with a cold and came home with lung cancer.

The Third Traveler's Tale: Marilyn

We had gone out of town for a wedding and came home on a Sunday night. The next day was Halloween. I had to work late that day, so I asked my husband to come home early so that he could give out the trick-or-treat candy when the children came to the house. The next morning, I heard him on the telephone canceling his meetings with clients for the day. I thought this was a little unusual. When he got off the phone, he just looked at me without saying anything. I said, "What's up?" He said, "Oh, I don't think it's much, but I've had a little pain in my chest for quite a while now." He said that his pain was never really sharp, but that it never went away completely either. "I felt it last night when I was giving the kids their candy." I thought that he was having a heart attack.

We immediately went to the hospital. After three full days of testing in the cardiac unit, they told my husband that his heart was fine. When our friends came to visit him in the hospital, they were so relieved to see how good he looked that they made the whole thing into a joke. The doctors sent him home, but they didn't want to give up without having a definite diagnosis. Just before Thanksgiving, after more weeks of tests, they saw a shadow on his lung. "A shadow," we thought, "can't be any big deal." Actually, the radiologist took us into his office and put the pictures up on the viewing box. "I think you're in really good shape," he said. "You see how the tumor is self-contained? This is something we can handle." My husband and I skipped out of the hospital like children. "It's nothing. It's just a nicely contained shadow. They can take care of that, easily."

A week later, the oncologist told us a very different story. We learned that my husband had the most aggressive form of lung cancer there is. "It will go through your body like a freight train," the oncologist told us. I will never be the same again after hearing those words.

The Fourth Traveler's Tale: Carlotta

My partner was feeling nauseated and vomiting a lot, so she and I went to the doctor. That was May. When we told the doctors that she and I had gone to Jamaica the previous March, they decided that she must have picked up an intestinal bug on the island. They started treating her for a tropical parasitic infection. I let that treatment go on even though I knew that she had been sick months before we ever went to Jamaica. Still, when the doctors said "parasite," I was willing to believe it.

When the treatment was not doing any good and she was getting worse, I called the doctor myself. I knew we weren't telling the doctor the entire story. I said, "When she is throwing up, it looks like diarrhea to me." When the doctor heard that, he called her back into the office that very day. They took some pictures, and that's when they found her stomach cancer.

The Fifth Traveler's Tale: Stephen

My wife had had a nagging cold for about six weeks, so we went to her doctor. Her physician said that her tests didn't show anything except that she was a little anemic. My wife took the iron he prescribed, but she still felt sick. We thought there must be some other fancy drug that would take care of her persistent cold and the feeling of malaise. She went back to the doctor. We were confident that they would get this thing figured out, sooner or later. Still, weeks went by and she wasn't feeling any better.

I came home from work late that fateful afternoon. My wife was sitting at the dining room table with our two young children. There was the usual mayhem with the children when I walked in. Nothing was unusual. Nothing was out of place. I walked into the kitchen with my wife before the usual dinner time download of information. She said to me, "I've got to talk to you about the blood test I had today.

Something's not right." I remember I was just reaching into the refrigerator at that moment to get a bottle of juice. She said, "They told me there are plasma cells in my blood." It just froze me instantly because I know what that usually means: plasma cell leukemia, which is a form of multiple myeloma.

As I clutched the juice bottle, I could only think that this was bad. At the same time, I told myself, "Do not look like this is serious. Think about this before you say anything." I didn't ask her for any further information, which of course was odd behavior on my part. She must have seen that.

That night I was lonely and unhappy. My only comfort was the statistics of the situation: The odds of this actually being multiple myeloma were very, very small. That gave me little comfort, however, because I knew in my heart that she was no longer in the normal statistical pool, now that she told me this information.

The next day, we were scheduled for a meeting with the doctors and a bone marrow biopsy. Everything I saw, everything I felt went from bad to worse. When we went into the hematology/oncology waiting room that next day, they gave us a menu of diseases for us to check off my wife's diagnosis. I went down the list and saw that there was nothing good there. They were all malignancies. That was the first time we had to confront just how bad it was. But, since I didn't know for sure what she had, I shut off the worst guesses. I said to my wife (but I was really talking to myself), "Let's just see how the tests turn out."

They did a bone marrow aspirate and told us to go off and have lunch and then to come back in a few hours. I recognized for the first time, as we sat in a little restaurant near the hospital, that the rest of the world is already different from ours. They're living, and we're facing who knows what. Sitting in this environment where normal life was going on all around us, I thought it would just be too melodramatic for us to go back to have the doctor tell us that my wife had a fatal disease.

We had a normal conversation over lunch: children, plans for the summer, work.

When we went back, the big cheese doctor came into the office in his white coat. He didn't make any eye contact. He didn't say hello. The second he walked into the room, he said, "I have bad news. It's multiple myeloma."

My wife doesn't understand biology and she doesn't care about statistics. She is not interested in hard facts. She relies on her instinct. She feels how things are from how people talk about them. In other words, she got the doctor's message. She got to the conclusion by a different route from mine, but she probably got a stronger sense of what the true situation was.

When bad news comes, it hits me, I feel a chill, and then I think that this is really going to feel bad, when the reality of the news hits home. I can't remember a damn thing after that. I completely cracked up. I can't remember feeling anything. I can't remember going home, being home, dealing with the kids that day. She was calm, too calm. That was the last time we were OK together as husband and wife.

The Sixth Traveler's Tale: Sarah

I first saw a lump in November of 1992 right in the corner of my husband's eye. I said to him, "Oh my gosh. What is that? What if that's a tumor?" My husband and I both know that I'm a worrier and an alarmist. He had noticed the little bump earlier and decided that it was a pimple. I know that I'm an alarmist, but now I blame myself for not making him go to the doctor sooner.

We were living in England when the first signs of trouble showed up. The National Health Service doctors first diagnosed it as conjunctivitis. Four months later, when the "conjunctivitis" wasn't going away, they did a CT scan. Three weeks later we got the results. "Oh yes," they said, "it looks like something is in there after all. It looks like a growth." When we heard that, we decided that he would see a doctor back here in the US.

The American doctors realized right away that my husband had a tumor. The biopsy suggested that it was benign, although the growth was pretty spread out. It started in the lachrymal sac and then went into all the little nooks and crannies around his eye. "Good news," they said to me. "It is only precancerous." He had surgery.

I was pregnant and not feeling well at the time. I remember being worried and feeling so vulnerable. When I asked the doctor, "What if this is cancer?" he said to me, "You don't even have to think about that. That's nothing you should be worrying about." The surgery went well.

Two days after our daughter was born in October, my husband had a recurrence. This time I wasn't worried. I thought that they had just missed a little something and that they would just mop it up. The pathology was still benign.

We were back in England for a vacation, and he started having nosebleeds. I got worried again. A month before, he had had a very severe nosebleed. He may have had some others, too. We dismissed these nosebleeds as nothing serious. After all, everybody gets nosebleeds. Sometimes it was hard to stop the bleeding, but that's not so strange.

When we came back to the US, he was scheduled for another surgery. They did a little biopsy, and again I wasn't worried about it. Then one evening, after dinner, my husband said to me, "I got a phone call from the doctor today and the biopsy showed something called carcinoma in situ." They still called it "precancer," but it was starting to sound like cancer to us. We were really shaken at that point.

We had the surgery, and the pathology confirmed that he had some very rare form of cancer called inverted papilloma. They decided to do radiation therapy. The radiation doctor said to us—with exaggerated optimism, I thought—that my husband would definitely live to see our daughter's graduation from college. "Everything will be fine," he said.

My husband began having a number of sinus infections after that, and then he was hospitalized. Then the tumor came back in July, with more nosebleeds. The doctor called and asked us to meet him at his office on a Sunday morning. Those were our last days of being carefree, before the coming of the cancer. Even with all the signs directly before our eyes, and with my tendency to worry, we were still trying to put the best construction on what we were going through.

He had more operations. Now the surgeons didn't tell us exactly what they were going to do. After one of the operations, the resident said that they had removed "the whole ball of wax" this time. They took out the right side of his hard palate and all of the teeth on that side of his mouth. That was shocking.

From that following October to December he was having more nosebleeds. The biopsy showed more carcinoma in situ. They proposed treating with a laser to mop up some more. When we wanted a second opinion, we had to wait a few months for an appointment.

In the meantime, my husband was developing what looked to me like another bump. His mother and I were sure that we saw something, but he said there was nothing there. The doctor said there was nothing there. As we were driving down to New York for the appointment at Mt. Sinai, my husband said to me, "I'm just doing this for you. There's no reason for us to go down. I'm just doing this for you." I didn't say anything. I was thinking that I just wanted to hear the doctor in New York say that everything was OK. We got ourselves settled in the examining room. Then in walked the doctor. The first thing he said to my husband was "What's that bump on your face?"

I felt horrible. I felt that I hadn't been sure enough of what I had been seeing. It's hard when you live with someone and see him all the time. The changes are so gradual. When it was diagnosed as carcinoma in situ, it never entered my mind that it could get worse. It had stayed like that for quite a while. We never expected that it would turn into cancer.

There were more surgeries. This time the plastic surgeon said everything looked clean. That was October. We were elated. We had come through the worst times together and now we could put the whole thing behind us. Two weeks later, he had a little thing that looked iffy, so they biopsied it. The next day, he was in the chair having the stitches removed. He got a message that the other doctor wanted to see him right away.

My husband asked me to come with him. I was afraid that the tumor had come back, but I didn't think of anything worse. The doctor ushered us into an examining room. He shoved the MRI films into the light box and said, "This is serious." In three months, a huge tumor grew to threaten my husband's eye. It was now frankly cancer. We had gone from thinking that we had escaped to something worse than before.

Once it was called "cancer"—no longer just "precancer"—we stepped over a line that we could never recross. Up to that point, I could worry and still believe deep inside that worrying was just neurotic. When you hear "cancer," you know that you have something real to worry about.

It's like growing up for us. And it has made my children grow up. They live in a different world now. It is a real loss of innocence. It feels like someone or something can just come in and squash you. We felt blessed in a lot of ways, before this. Now I feel cursed. I am the daughter of concentration camp survivors, so I learned from my parents that we cannot take anything for granted. We cannot trust that good things will last or that rescues from disaster can happen without leaving terrible scars. There is research that if you destroy a spider's web, they can rebuild it. It's not exactly like the old one, but it is serviceable. If you keep destroying the web, each time it is less and less beautiful and less functional. After each step in the treatment, we put our lives back together, but each time a little less perfectly. Now I feel we will never go back to the perfect world we used to have. Now I feel like I am just sitting in the wreckage, trying to put it back together.

A *midrash* (one of the famous ancient Jewish commentaries on a biblical passage) explains that when God was making the world, something he was working on dropped and shattered. One of the obligations of an observant Jew is the *tikkun olam*, the effort to put the imperfect part of the world back together. I feel that cancer is one of those shards. I can't understand why this would happen. If this could happen, then God must not be omnipotent, and if he is, why is this happening?

The Seventh Traveler's Tale: Theresa

There was nothing heart-wrenching about it at all. It's just that one day, my life changed. Just like that. In the morning, my partner and I ran around as usual. We were just two women getting ready for work. I drove her to her office that day because her own car was in the shop. We said our customary good-bye and those last-minute exchanges of information before we plunged into the busy day that was ahead for each of us. We said good-bye again, and I drove myself to work.

At the end of the day, just before leaving work for the day, I checked my voice mail, and there was a message from the emergency room at the hospital near where my partner worked. The message was that I should call the hospital, but that "there is nothing urgent." It didn't strike me as odd that the *emergency room* would say that it wasn't urgent. I thought instead, "She probably got into a minor fender-bender and has no way to get home." I also didn't think at the time, "Wait a minute. *I* drove her to work today. She doesn't have her car." So I called the hospital with only mild curiosity about what they might want from me. The emergency room doctor said that my partner had had a seizure while she was at work, and that I "should come right away." From that moment to today, our life has never been the same. She had a brain tumor.

The Eighth Traveler's Tale: My Own

For our fifteenth summer together, Trudee and I were staying in our cottage—The Nautilus—on Sandy Neck, a large sandbar jutting out into Cape Cod Bay in the town of Barnstable. It was mid-July 1994, a few days before her forty-fifth birthday.

Our days on Sandy Neck that July were like all idyllic days there before. Friends, water, blue sky, boats, fish, volleyball, food, poker games for stakes nobody could mind losing, and the two of us together. To add to the magic of the place, our only access to The Nautilus was by boat. We would climb into our little runabout and motor across Barnstable Harbor. The trip took twenty minutes at most. In that short time, we left the real world behind.

The Nautilus was primitive by any measure: We had no electricity. The cottage had running water, but only cold water and only if someone remembered to run the gasoline pump that fed the elevated cistern that supplied water to the six cottages of the compound. The telephone in one of the outbuildings was to be used for only the most necessary communications with the outside world. There was indoor plumbing, but in another building about fifty yards away from our cottage.

We slept on the second floor of The Nautilus, just under the roof. One of my fondest memories of the place is of lying in bed and looking up at the time-seasoned golden wood of the bare rafters and the underside of the roofing boards. For a time during the century of that cottage's existence, it housed part of a children's camp, and those children penciled their names, dates, and opinions of the cook's skills. When the wind blew, the old wood of the windows rattled dully in their tracks with an oddly reassuring thump. The wind also whistled a series of banshee tones as it blew over the caps of the unused propane gas tanks behind The Nautilus. The cottage protected us. Through the little window at the head of the bed, we could look out at the ebb and flow of the twelve-foot Barnstable Harbor tide and the regular flashing of the green buoy light where the channel turned, just in front of our cottage.

The toilet arrangement at the cottage bears directly on our moment of discovery. Because the trip to the outbuilding and toilet was usually an unwelcome disruption of sweet sleep, at night we took to using a jug rather than trudge to the outside bathroom. And, like plucking the branch from the tree of disaster, one night of peeing in the jar marked the beginning of our encounter with cancer.

"Look at this," Trudee said, "that flavored iced tea I was drinking yesterday must have come through in my pee." Indeed, her urine had a slight reddish tinge. The next day she stopped drinking the iced tea and the reddish color went away. Her theory was confirmed. The next day, however, her urine was the color of deep claret, and we needed a new explanation.

Trudee made one of those infrequent telephone calls from the phone in the outbuilding. She called a urologist. "It's probably nothing," he said. "If you were twenty, I'd prescribe a course of antibiotics and have you call me if it didn't clear up. But maybe you should come in so I can take a look."

We packed up and went back to town. Innocents.

The unpleasantness of Trudee's examination defies description. It revealed the presence of two very small polyps hanging on slender stalks from the lining of her bladder. The urologist snipped a small piece of one of the polyps for biopsy. "They are so small," he said, "that I will have no trouble just snipping them off. It's really just an office procedure."

We agreed. Innocents.

To expedite matters, the urologist handed us the biopsy tissue in a small plastic container and suggested that we take it ourselves to the pathologist to save time. "Sure," we said, and off we went, threading our way through the hospital corridors to the pathology department. The young pathologist who opened the laboratory door was surprised to see us. "We never get to see whole people up here," he said. We delivered our small burden to him and went home.

In a day or so, the urologist had a tentative diagnosis: transitional cell carcinoma of the bladder. Although that sounded bad to us, the urologist assured us that there were only those two little blebs and that he could remove them easily. There was nothing to be too upset about. Innocents. We did some chores in town—got Trudee's glasses from the optician, renewed her driver's license at the Registry, treated ourselves to a Dim Sum lunch, and then had the car serviced.

We went back to Sandy Neck. Except for the fact that Trudee had an appointment the following week for the minor procedure (in a hospital this time) to remove the polyps from her bladder, every-thing was fine. Innocents. Just to be on the safe side, however, the urologist ordered some simple x-rays, "just to rule out some things." "Sure," we said, "might as well rule some things out." We went back to Sandy Neck.

The day we came back to town for the x-rays was another of those fine Cape Cod summer days. It was early August. The x-ray was no big deal. Everything about it was familiar and routine. Until the technician said to Trudee that he could not find her left kidney on the screen. He what? "Oh, there it is," he said. "It's pushed way up from its normal position." Then he got very quiet. A later CT scan confirmed the situation.

It was the urologist who explained that a large mass was shoving T's kidney aside. "What kind of mass?" we asked. That would require more tests. Innocents. Meanwhile, the biopsy came back with an unclear diagnosis.

We were sent to another physician, a diagnostic radiologist, who had a new CT scan machine. There were only three of these in the entire United States. It was an open CT device so that a physician could stand inside with the patient and use the image from the CT scan to guide the biopsy needle. Yes, Trudee would need another biopsy, this time of the large mass.

We met with this physician to discuss the biopsy. His excitement about his new machine far outweighed his concern for us. In fact, we were slowly beginning to recognize that the medical experts were intensifying their efforts. We were alarmed, but vaguely. The biopsy was drawn. And we waited. And waited. Our lives came to a stop.

A few days later, we had an idea. Trudee worked at the hospital and had access to the computer system that contained, among other things, patient records. With her password, we could sit at my desk and have my computer dial up the hospital computer (all this was perfectly legal). We had done this before, once or twice, when Trudee had had minor medical problems. It was intriguing to see how the medical information was packaged for internal medical use.

After negotiating a few computer menus, we got to Trudee's medical record. Our experience of the past week or so was com-pressed to a few paragraphs of medical jargon. We sat at my desk staring at the computer screen, thinking, "Oh, finally, we are going to find out what's what."

Well, not quite. But what we discovered was bad enough.

Tentative diagnosis: Lymphoma.

"It's like reading my own death warrant," Trudee said.

We sat stunned. We had no buffer of a physician standing between the harsh reality and our fears. We were alone. We hugged in silence and turned off the computer. That was the last time we went to the computer for information about Trudee's diagnosis or treatment. We had looked too directly at the reality of what we were facing.

Not since I was three years old have I heard myself make the sounds that came out of me that day. I had to reach awkwardly over the arm of my desk chair to reach Trudee while we held each other and sobbed. No, "sob" makes it sound too genteel. Trudee held me tight as I howled out of control. I can still feel how the chair arm dug into my ribs and the dull pain as each violent intake of my breath pushed me harder against the chair. I was kneeling across the chair with my head in Trudee's lap. Trudee cried quietly and more or less collapsed onto me collapsed onto her. We stayed in that position for a long time before we eventually cried ourselves out.

Fear had an unexpected effect on us. For first time in our life together, we both could feel the fragility of what we had. That recognition filled us with mutual tenderness and delicacy. We became selfless. In that instant, the boundaries between us dissolved. It comforted me to help Trudee with her pain. And, if I may speak for her, it eased her own burden to be comforting me. Intensely happy events, such as the birth of a baby, may be similar when we take pleasure in another person's happiness. But happiness is infectious, anyhow. It was a profound surprise to learn that we were not alone in our fear and anguish either.

That moment initiated us into our new life. That moment of discovery and the few days that followed contained the germs of all the dramas that would eventually be played out in the rest of our time with cancer.

As it turned out, lymphoma was not the final diagnosis. In fact, when we finally learned the true diagnosis, lymphoma looked good. Lymphoma can be treated with some success. What Trudee had, the physicians told us, was known as leiomyosarcoma. The condition is very rare, with no more than six thousand cases a year in the United States. Most of these are leiomyosarcomas of the extremities. Trudee's was located in the back of the space that contains her stomach, intestines, and liver. Those organs were not being invaded, but like her kidney, they were being pushed aside by this growing mass.

We met with the physicians early in August to discuss the future. What treatment was available? What were the chances of success? What was success? Trudee and I made it clear from the outset that we needed to hear the whole truth. "The situation is difficult enough," we said to them, "that if we couldn't believe that we were getting the whole truth, the uncertainty would just make things harder for us. We need the straight scoop."

Having made that little speech, I took a deep breath to regain control of my voice and asked them, "So how long does Trudee have to live?" "One-third of all patients survive three to six months," the doctor replied. In our shock, we didn't ask about the other two-thirds.

"Is there treatment?"

"Many treatments are possible, but there is no guaranteed effective treatment." Again, in our shock we didn't ask whether any of the treatments held at least a reasonable chance of being effective.

"Does this form of cancer metastasize?" Trudee asked.

"Yes."

"To the bone?" she asked.

"Rarely."

"To the brain?"

"Rarely."

Those were Trudee's worst fears. So, in a strange way, there was some relief.

She was far ahead of me in thinking through the implications of our new life.

When we went back to Sandy Neck in mid-August we were changed people. During the weeks before, we kept what we were going through to ourselves. We knew so little hard information that it seemed pointless to say anything. It would just alarm people without giving them anything concrete to deal with. After our later meetings with the physicians, we did have the hard information. This time we deliberately kept our news secret. Even in the intimate setting of Sandy Neck itself, where we were more like a large family, we told no one. We needed time to deal with our own fears before we could accept those of others.

The Geography at the Border

New arrivals appeared at the inn while our little knot of travelers was exchanging stories. They sat off by themselves for the most part, the newcomers, but I could see them eyeing us nervously. Not joining us, but watching. I could also see that while we were talking, other groups ahead of us gathered themselves together and left the inn. Alone, in small groups, reluctantly, they departed. Their red-rimmed eyes still burned from the smoke that filled the rooms of the inn. So, in a strange way, there was even a bit of comfort in leaving the inn at the border crossing. The inn gave little shelter, nor was it meant to.

Just beyond the exit from the inn, the nondescript gateway into the cancer world now lies in front of us. It is little more than a movable barrier, like the gate at a rural railroad crossing, that gives access to a small patch of ground—the waiting area inside a kind of no-man's land. A few stone and metal benches are arranged in rows in this waiting area. But the main feature of the waiting area is the set of aisles, hand-rails made of pipes, leading from the benches forward to a small building with five windows, and a narrow metal counter in front of each window. Behind three of the windows are men in uniform who dispense the entry forms that are required for passing through the gate.

People line up in the three aisles leading to the windows that have border guards, get their entry forms, return to the benches in the waiting area to fill out their forms, and then get in line again to present their completed forms at the window. Surprisingly, even with the current of people moving toward the windows and the counter-current of people returning from the windows, there is little shoving. Even when the three guards decide to change windows arbitrarily, which they do frequently, the mass of applicants just reforms itself in the newly activated aisles. A similar gate is visible at the other side of the waiting area.

We spend an inordinate amount of time in the waiting area between the gates. We can see a little of what we guess must be the cancer world beyond the second gate. We look at the other people sitting in the waiting room, preparing for their CT scans and MRIs. Some of those people are quite sick. Some are anxious. Some have the tolerant look of veterans who have been in that waiting room before. They don't mind the passage of time. Some are alone, others speak a few words to companions who fidget beside them. One of the companions is reading a six-month-old *Time* magazine. The pages have been softened by so much nervous handling that they make no sound when they are turned. Most of the partners sit doing nothing, lost in their own thoughts. Except for the border guards who patrol this territory, no one speaks more than a few perfunctory words. In contrast, the border guards are openly jocular with each other. They chatter about the food in the cafeteria, the long work hours, the computer system, what they did last weekend.

From time to time, the border guards may say something informative or friendly to the patients. They almost never acknowledge the presence of the equally nervous person accompanying the patient. As a result, the companions in this way station sit like fifth wheels. They find it difficult to penetrate their partner's anxiety, so the two of them sit side by side in very different universes. They are of only passing interest to the border guards, too. Occasionally, one partner will catch the eye of another sitting there, and there may be the momentary thickening of a common bond. The next person is called into the MRI room and the partnerships are thrust two-by-two into their own separate adventures.

Time doesn't exactly stop in the gateway to the cancer world; it gets distorted. Each moment seems to hang heavy, but then we realize with a start that we have been in this no-man's land for more than three hours. It was the same yesterday. We go from one appointment to another for diagnostic tests. We work hard to help the doctors make a diagnosis. They, too, work hard. But they seem to know already the very thing we dread learning. Possible diagnoses are floated pending further tests, but the tentative diagnoses are often too frightening to accept. We still think that the next round of tests will show that the condition is nothing too serious. In the meantime, we wait.

Something else happens, too. We become fascinated by the process itself. The technology available at the border crossing is truly amazing. At one station, we see pictures of the most intimate details of our partner's body. The information is so intrinsically interesting, in fact, that we forget a little about why it is being shown to us.

Then, without much fanfare, we have slipped through the second gate and have entered the cancer world. The doctors say, "We are now pretty sure that you have . . . ." That's it. The weeks of tests are summarized in one fateful sentence.

Trudee and I sat in the doctor's office and held each other's hands. There was nothing else to do. We didn't cry until we got home. It was my first awkward attempt at playing the role of the cancer partner.

And How Are You Doing?

And the seas of pity lie
Locked and frozen in each eye.
—*W.H. Auden,* In Memory of W.B. Yeats

*W*hy is the following scene so difficult for cancer partners? You are talking with an acquaintance—someone familiar enough to know about your partner's cancer, but not someone with whom you would ordinarily share the intimate details of your life. After talking about some commonplace things, the conversation turns to polite questions about how your partner is feeling or how the chemotherapy is going. You answer as vaguely and as briefly as possible, already feeling the muscles of your face tightening into a fixed and neutral expression. You would like to change the subject or, better yet, say good-bye and leave. Before you can escape, however, there is a momentary hitch in the conversation. The asker's voice modulates to a tone of careful concern that paradoxically avoids betraying any real feeling before confronting you with the question that disarms and disturbs most cancer partners: "And how are *you* doing?"

Talking with other cancer partners made me realize that most cancer partners are put off by this seemingly innocent question. A woman I met in the cancer world tells me that she hates the question and always answers, "I'm hanging in there. I'm OK." This is only the empty shell of a response, of course, but it is often enough to extricate her from what she finds a terribly awkward situation. I responded with the same painful evasion.

I think we can learn some important things about what it means to be a cancer partner from the almost universal discomfort this question generates. The pain, I think, comes from the awareness we all have of how the vagueness of the answer contradicts the gritty reality of our lives in the cancer world. In a sense, we catch ourselves in a lie when we give a simple, evasive answer. Deception in this case is easier than telling the truth. Our discomfort is the price we pay for that deception.

Another cancer partner whose husband has esophageal cancer gives a glimpse of what lies behind her breezy answer that she is OK. "It's not my personality to run around in a frenzy, so it was very bizarre for me to feel my heart pounding, day and night. I remember walking into the grocery store and looking at the food at the deli counter and realizing that I was just seeing colors and textures. I was not seeing food. Because of my husband's esophageal cancer, I felt bad to be eating anything when he couldn't eat at all. So, if someone asked me how I was doing, I would have to say truthfully that I was in a panic all the time and I was starving myself to death. Would anybody want to hear that? No. Instead I just told them that I was doing OK."

A man I met whose wife has metastatic breast cancer also gives the general public a sanitized response to the question. "In our family, we have been in an almost continual state of extra tension for more than two years," he says. "It's been really rotten. My mother-in-law suffered a slow, lingering, horrible death from breast cancer, and my wife took care of her. My own father died of cancer, my sister has breast cancer, and now my wife has it. I feel like I am surrounded by cancer. In addition to the cancer, our two teenage boys fight constantly with each other, and my wife will not discipline them. I'm sure that she wants to be remembered by the boys as a good, warm mother. Automatically that means I am the bad guy. What can I do? It really bothers me when people ask how I'm doing because all this bad stuff almost comes out. I don't really want it to. I feel so stuck. I feel so unhappy. I feel so alone. I feel like I am at my wit's end. I don't want to be at work. I don't want to be at home. I don't want to be alone. If someone I meet in the corridor at work asks me how I am doing, I can't open up all this."

I'm sure that the person who asks "And how are *you* doing?" really believes that asking is a show of support for us cancer partners. But the person who asks that question is invariably an outsider merely peeking in at the cancer world. By asking the question, such a casual inquirer makes a brief excursion into a highly charged and sometimes unpredictable emotional atmosphere. Like anyone visiting a world with its own complex rules of etiquette and social customs, the outsider who wanders into the cancer world is almost sure to blunder. Although well intentioned, the visitor is often slightly off the mark.

Perhaps this critique of such an innocent-sounding question sounds uncharitable. People do want to help and many are truly interested in how we are. Trudee and I got a great deal of good-natured, loving, positive, and clear support from our friends and family. These people were very good at striking just the right tone in expressing their support. They knew how to express their solidarity with us without also attaching emotional strings. Sometimes, however, we found ourselves dealing with the fears and neuroses of the person asking the question—anxieties expressed under the pretext of concern for us. I think this is one of the reasons the question is so off-putting. Instead of joining us in the cancer world by saying outright that this is a dreadful experience for them as well as for us, these people ask the question in such a way that we are forced to deal with *their* fears, even as they pretend to be concerned about us.

The question, "And how are *you* doing?" is the cancer world equivalent of asking someone who has just returned from a trip, "So how was it?" You can answer, "The trip was fantastic," which is what the questioner expects to hear—even wants to hear—and leave it at that. Or you can go into the real details of the trip, which may surprise the questioner.

In easier times, Trudee and I traveled to foreign cities. When we got home, we would tell friends about the small adventures we had buying forty bottles of red and green salsa in a supermarket in Mexico or wandering lost in a maze of small streets and back alleys in Paris. Once, we successfully avoided getting shaken down for a fifty-dollar bribe by a traffic policeman in Bratislava. Another time, we jumped on the wrong bus coming back from a mammoth flea market on the outskirts of Budapest and were led back to our hotel by an old man who spoke only Turkish. In recounting these adventures to those friends who wondered what museums we visited (none), or what well-known restaurants we patronized (only a few), or what itinerary we planned before leaving home (we didn't), our stories often fell flat. The point of the adventure was lost on them. On the other hand, people who themselves had stories about knocking around in hardware stores in Portugal or being asked to read a few pages of *Willie Wonka and the Chocolate Factory* in English to uncomprehending villagers in Vietnam enjoyed hearing our adventures, and understood them. Stories of our travels in the cancer world are similar to our other travel tales. People who have felt the force of their own travels (originally the same word as "travails") know how to ask the questions that reveal the depth of their own fellow feeling. Those people wouldn't ask "And how are *you* doing?"—at least not in the same way.

Crossing the border into the cancer world changes something in us so that old ways of talking politely no longer suffice. Those who have not crossed the border can easily offend us by asking a conventional question—they rarely get the tone right, and not asking is just as bad. But the main source of the difficulty must be in us if so many cancer partners feel discomfort when asked this question. Something terribly complicated must be going on psychologically if such an innocuous question makes us feel so bad.

The question "And how are *you* doing?" can make cancer partners wince for several reasons. It is worth our while to think a bit about why we are so sensitive to this question. After all, many people who ask the question are trying to help. Although their intentions may be good—and we certainly need all the support we can get—something goes wrong. Perhaps, then, we should look to ourselves.

We Envy the Asker's Innocence

One reason the question bothers cancer partners is that a gulf exists between us and those who ask the question. People who ask "And how are *you* doing?" are calling to us in the cancer world from their safe place across the border. Just asking such a naïve question emphasizes the boundary between their world and ours. "Those people know nothing about our situation," one cancer partner says. The gulf between their world and hers was so obvious, she thought, that even if she wanted to, "I couldn't really get them to understand what my life is really like." Even if she could somehow get them to understand, she concludes, "I don't think they want to hear my real emotions."

We may also envy the askers their innocence. Like the rabbi who replied when asked why he always answered a question with another question, "So how else should I answer?," so should we probably answer this question with another question. "Compared with what? Compared with the pre-cancer life, I'm doing terribly. Compared with yesterday when Trudee vomited all day, I'm doing a lot better."

But that response has a nuance that innocent people who haven't traveled in the cancer world may have trouble understanding. "The real issue," says another cancer partner, "is that the people who ask really don't know what you are going through. They ask that question on the basis of the easiest assumptions about what life with cancer is like. If they really know us, they can see for themselves that living with cancer is very difficult." The single sentence, "Today was a pretty good day" has all the pathos of a full-length tragedy if we know how to read it. Wouldn't it be nice, we think to ourselves, to be so blissfully unaware of the cancer life that a person has to ask!

Meanwhile, we want our support to come from someone who doesn't need to ask but who has already made the effort of looking around in the cancer world. What feels like a casual visit is therefore a little offensive. We are like poor inhabitants of a slum in some foreign city who watch the tour buses roll by on their way to a local attraction. We want to ignore the comfortable tourists in their air-conditioned buses, but we can't ignore them if they are asking us where we got our beautiful hats or how many children we have. A casual visit to the cancer world won't substitute for real travel there.

We Are Annoyed by a Conventional Question in an Unconventional Setting

The question is also grating to many cancer partners because it is such a conventional question, but it is asked in a completely unconventional context. Life within the cancer world has its own social rules—adaptations of some of the baggage that we carried across the border from innocence to cancer. Like settlers in a new land who adapt the familiar old styles of architecture or cooking to the realities of what is available in the new land, we cancer partners establish new ways of living in the cancer world on the basis of what we did before entering it. To do this, whether we are aware of the process or not, we test the usefulness of those social conventions that were almost perfectly transparent in the old world of innocence. In the old world, when life was comfortable and easy, we rarely questioned our deepest assumptions. We took easy refuge behind euphemisms to ease difficult social situations. The formulas of polite discourse normally served us well; there was little need to get to the heart of things in casual conversation. In the cancer world, however, we are forced to look at things we can no longer ignore. People all around us live with fear and pain. People die. We adapt to the new realities of the cancer world or we become a calcified parody of the figure that used to be us in the old world.

We Resent Other People's Pity

Cancer partners also usually hear condescension and pity filling the brief pause in the conversation that comes just before the question "And how are *you* doing?" The look in the other person's eyes is a little too searching. The face is too firmly set in an expression of sympathy. The instinct to pick up a bird with a broken wing is a little too obvious. Cancer partners are sustained by other people's concern (literally, a mingling together), and it helps us share our unease, apprehension, and fear. Concern like this depends on a personal tie between us. But most cancer partners I met are made very uncomfortable by pity (literally, piety). Being the object of someone's concern is far different from being the object of someone's pity. After all, who wants to feel pitiful? Self-pity is one of the private demons we cancer partners fight all the time.

We Are Reminded that Our Partner Is Separate

Separation lurks in the background of nearly everything we do in the cancer world. The question "And how are *you* doing?" insinuates that very separation between the partners we are striving to minimize. "A lot of the time I don't feel that I am my wife's *partner*," says one cancer partner, "but rather that we *both* have the cancer. There are times when it is hard to distinguish my role from hers. That is one of the complicated parts of the experience: that you are watching the person who is closest to you struggle with the cancer in a very concrete sense while, at the same time, you have the same cancer in some figurative sense." The question "And how are *you* doing?" shifts the focus of attention to only one of us rather than to the partnership itself. People don't mean to do this when they ask the question, but it feels like a dividing wedge between the two partners, just when we are struggling to stay together.

Cancer partners are very sensitive to anything that might separate us, even symbolically. A woman whose husband underwent a complicated biopsy for his throat cancer says that the question generates the same feeling in her as when she telephoned her husband's brother in another city. "I told him that the biopsy showed some kind of cancer and that my husband would need more tests before they would know just what kind of cancer he had, and how to treat it. Then his brother said the strangest thing to me, 'Oh, I'm so sorry. I hate to think of you all by yourself up there.' That was such a funny remark. I said to him, 'I'm not alone. I have my husband.' The question 'And how are *you* doing?' brings back that same feeling of being isolated and separated from my husband."

We Know It Is Not a Real Question

Often times, the people who ask the question don't really want to know so much *how* you are doing, but rather *that* you are doing OK. By telling them that you are getting along OK, you are saying that there is no need to worry. "When I take the question at all seriously, I realize that the question is horribly intrusive," explains one cancer partner. "I think they really want to know if I have enough people to talk to, whether I am doing things for myself, that I know how to find support for myself. When I just say that I'm OK, I know that 'OK' is an abbreviation for a much more complicated answer, but I usually can't give the real answer to most people. The real answer would blow them away. 'OK' means for me, as a character says in one of Jane Smiley's novels, 'I'm still recognizable to myself. I haven't gone crazy. I'm still sane.' But in truth there's a pretty strong sense that we're walking on very thin ice. Somebody in our family could break through at any moment. We're holding on for today. Even that answer is a struggle with the truth because I know that we are not really managing at all."

We Share a Private Language in the Cancer World

Trudee and I worked out our own comfort levels with the changes we were going through and with our own ways of dealing with her illness. In doing so, we developed our own vernacular. The cancer vernacular simply extended the dialect that our richly intertwined life had created. Another life would have created a different dialect, but cancer created this one. Like other dialects, the patois of the cancer world can be imitated by outsiders, but it cannot be generated with all its welter of associations.

Sometimes, the cancer was familiar enough to take a joke. One night when Trudee was too worn out to accept a friend's invitation to dinner, she said to me, in an uncharacteristic outburst, "I don't think I can get through that dinner." She fantasized about calling our hosts and saying to them in her sweetest manner, "I'm so sorry we won't be able to come to dinner, but I'm just shot through with cancer tonight." We laughed, finished getting dressed, and went to dinner.

You can't recreate the cancer vocabulary on the spot and teach it to the innocent who pose that difficult question "And how are *you* doing?" Between us, Trudee and I could make the necessary accommodations for the cancer that she called her "evil twin." Talking this way with most other people was difficult because even close friends were not living on such intimate terms with the cancer. It's not all that different from other spoken and physical intimacies between two people in love—the private jokes that need no more than a casual reference by their abbreviated label ("windshield wipers," for us, for example) to raise a smile and a giggle, the touch of the fingers that says, "Oy, did we ask for this?"

We Feel Our Ambivalence

The question "And how are *you* doing?" also makes it clear that the cancer partner can act as a double agent living simultaneously in two worlds: the harsh cancer world and the pleasant old world. It is a difficult choice—but it is a choice, after all—to take on the cancer life as a partner. But our decision is fraught with ambivalence, and the question from an outsider makes us face all the unpleasant tension of unresolved ambivalence. The outside world often fails to recognize this tension, however, and may minimize the cancer partner's role. We choose to stay in this difficult world, but we don't like the choice.

As active partners in the cancer world, we play a role equal to that of our partner with cancer. Others may not understand the stresses that come with that role. Says one cancer partner: "I don't like the question because, if it is *my* friends who are asking, I wonder why they aren't asking first about how *I* am doing. If they are *my* friends and they see *me*, I want them to ask about *me* first. The way in which they ask the question, after spending a lot of time talking about *her*, makes me feel like I am second fiddle. I know it sounds selfish, but my partner's cancer is affecting me, too. I am not just a second fiddle. I want other people to recognize that this is my life that is going down the drain with hers."

We Defend Our Defenses

The question "And how are *you* doing?" is also discomforting because it threatens the defensive bulwarks that we build for ourselves. Denial and other defenses help get us through the daily pressures in the cancer world. Repression (a psychological process that is normally outside our awareness) and suppression (our more deliberate effort to put something out of mind) operate in different balances at different times. These are normal psychological defenses that help protect us when the reality before us is intolerably painful. Defenses like these allow us emotional time off. The intrusive question, "And how are *you* doing?" strips away some of those handy defenses. "When people ask about my husband, and then turn to me with that question," says a cancer partner, "I just about fall apart. I can't respond because I have such a big lump in my throat. Their direct question forces me to acknowledge that this whole thing could be having an effect on me. 'Something must be very wrong,' I think, 'or they wouldn't be asking me in that way.' At the same time, I am also thinking, 'My husband has cancer. How am I supposed to be? How do you think I'm doing?' I want to scream at them, 'I'm doing terribly!'"

Another cancer partner echoes this sentiment. "People usually ask me that question when my partner and I are at a social gathering. I am relaxing, away from my partner and away from her cancer for a few moments. I am doing my darndest to maintain the façade—for myself and for everyone else—that things are still OK for us. Then suddenly, when my guard is down, I am trapped by someone asking the question that brings me back to that horribly painful focus of our lives. I feel constantly like we are both just dangling by a thread. Having someone ask that question only makes the thread thinner for that moment."

We can play the role of the cancer partner largely because our defenses allow us to focus on everything *but* the frightening and painful parts of the cancer world. The defenses make it possible to get through days of waiting for test results, trying to encourage our partners to eat or drink, or helping with the countless personal necessities that illness or weakness make difficult. We get through the day by evading the recognition that there is something really odd (and threatening) about having a hospital bed in the living room and an oxygen tank in the corner.

So How *Are* You Doing?

One way of dealing with the emotional life of the cancer partnership is to take no emotional role at all. One cancer partner tries not to let his feelings out. "If I'm alone, that's one thing," he says, "but I wouldn't want my feelings to come out when I'm with my wife. I'm sure that she has cried many times by herself. But when I'm with her, I think that my job is to be strong for her. That's not easy for me to do because her cancer is a hard situation for me to get a handle on."

Crying together, on the other hand, is good sign of how well the cancer partnership is faring. First of all, it is a strong signal to get your attention. To suppress that signal is like turning off the smoke detector in your house. A fire could be smoldering and about to burst into flames while you are totally unaware of the danger. Crying is a recognition of the sad threat that has loomed into our lives. Crying together is something more than the emotional awareness of what is happening, it is a willingness to share that awareness. Sharing the sadness in such an elemental way—holding each other and letting the tears stream down—makes it clear, as only such "animal" behavior can do, that we are in the cancer world together. That emotional solidarity is the foundation on which all the good qualities of the cancer partnership are built.

Even harder than crying together is the effort to put the sad threat into words. Talking together and with other people is the ultimate sign of how the cancer partnership is surviving the rigors of travel in the cancer world. Talk that is just idle words is pointless. But talk that gives expression to the tears is invaluable. It is one of the early steps in finding meaning in our otherwise desolate experiences of the cancer world.

The other side of the experience—a sign of how badly we are doing—is how strongly we feel trapped by circumstances. We must acknowledge that we have lost important parts of our own private lives. But we also must acknowledge that we trap ourselves. It is hard for us to get out of the cancer world, and we are sometimes afraid to try the freedom of separating ourselves even the slightest bit from the rigors of the cancer life. We cancer partners act as if our role requires constant vigilance. We fear that if we let down our guard for an instant, something will happen even more dreadful than what we've already gone through. This obsessiveness is different from *wanting* to spend as much time as possible with the person we love. This is a kind of magical thinking that makes us to do things that we recognize are against our own best interests—and are probably contrary to what our partner would want us to do, as well—yet we do them anyway. Sometimes we cannot take a break, of course. But there are many other times when we can, but we choose not to.

I had trouble finding quick escapes from the cancer life. The day Trudee and I entered the cancer world, I stopped playing the piano, for example. Admittedly, this is not the equivalent of Artur Rubenstein or Thelonius Monk giving up the piano, but playing the piano was something I enjoyed. Not playing left a small emptiness in my life. I especially enjoyed the half-hour alone at home before Trudee came from work, which, in our old life, was a time when I could bang on the piano without inhibitions or self-consciousness. Only Hannah, our aging Chesapeake Bay retriever, was there to listen and criticize— something she rarely did. Whenever she heard me pull the bench out from under the piano, Hannah would lope into the living room and settle down on the rug.

After Trudee got sick, she would sometimes ask me why I wasn't playing anymore, and I would give her some half answer that was more an evasion than a response. The true reason for my not playing was that Trudee was now around the house all the time. Since the piano was in the living room, I became self-conscious about playing with Trudee as a captive audience. She tried telling me that she liked hearing me play. She couldn't convince me otherwise.

A woman who loved playing the flute similarly stopped playing when her husband was diagnosed. "It no longer felt right to play the flute while my husband lay there with his brain filling with aggressive, metastatic tumors," she says. It is one thing to be light-hearted together in confronting the cancer demons; it is quite a different thing to be the only light-hearted one while your partner with the cancer is suffering. Meanwhile, cancer partners also feel the finitude of time as never before; it is a finite commodity, fearfully measured in unusually short increments. This forces the painful choice on cancer partners to invest that precious resource carefully. Spend time on the two of us, or just on me? Investment in ourselves is always hard. Playing the flute or the piano for a few minutes seems like a small thing, but at the time it feels unpleasantly selfish.

Escaping the Role

Clearly we occasionally need to take a break from the cancer partner role in order to protect ourselves. Yet as the following stories make clear, the price of "escape" is often too high. Many of us attempt it once and decide it isn't worth the risks. Eventually, if we are lucky, we learn that although there is no escape, we are not trapped either. Escape would be a return to the pre-cancer life, but that is no longer possible.

Working to Defeat Cancer: Steven's Story

Steven is a scientist who works on cancer-related research. His wife has multiple myeloma. For him, his work is both an escape from his role as cancer partner and its deepest expression. "The fact that I work in this field has created a lot more tension because there is no moment when I don't feel that I should be doing something in the lab or in the library to help figure this thing out," he says. "The strain is almost unbearable. I am working on a personal test for my wife's kind of cancer, designed to detect her particular form of the cancer. If we succeed, we might be able to create a specific treatment for her. My wife feels that this research might lead to something that will save her. The double edge is that if it doesn't, she'll wonder what this was all about. I will wonder, too, whether I should have been doing all that work in the lab or whether I should have been at home with her. She appreciates the work in the lab, but she thinks I am not doing enough for her emotionally. I am beginning to wonder whether I am taking the easier path here—dealing with the challenges of lab technique rather than the emotional realities at home."

Father and Son: Don's Story

As part of his son's scouting experience, one cancer partner and his wife decided that father and son would go on a fifty-mile canoe trip exploring a lake in a remote part of northern Maine. His wife's condition seemed pretty stable at the time, and she encouraged her husband to go on the trip, saying it would make her happy to see the two men in her life working out plans for the expedition. As the day of their departure approached, however, she and her husband both got nervous about whether the separation was such a good idea. "We started to realize how remote the lake was, and how totally out of touch with each other we would be," he says. "The cancer made everything different for us. We started to cling to each other more than we had ever done before." To allay her fears and to give himself some peace of mind, he set up a tag-team of friends and relatives who would come in a couple of times a day to prepare meals, check on her, and keep her company. On the second day of the canoe trip, she was admitted to the hospital with terrible pain in her right rib, where the cancer had metastasized. Meanwhile, the man didn't know any of this until he and his son came home a week later. "The whole experience made me very reluctant to try any more outings. In fact, that was the last time I took any time off for myself."

My Own Escape

My own experience in getting away was similar. Trudee had just started her first cycle of chemotherapy. In this experimental protocol, called "high-dose ICE," she was given a combination of chemotherapy agents. Studies had shown that the standard chemotherapy for leiomyosarcoma wasn't very successful. Any one of the drugs would have made her feel sick, and she got high doses of all three. The hope was that this would deal a knockout blow to the growing tumors. "Why not give high-dose ICE a try?" we thought.

Some time before Trudee was diagnosed, a friend had invited me to go sailing with him on Chesapeake Bay that early autumn. We would take his boat across the bay and then go gunkholing up the little rivers that feed into the bay. I could stay for the entire two weeks of his trip or come along for part of the trip. He just needed to know how long I would stay. The other part of the deal was that once I was there, I had to stay because he needed me to serve as crew.

It seemed incredibly selfish to go sailing while Trudee was in the throes of her chemotherapy. Her first experience with the high-dose ICE protocol was pretty rough. I didn't want to leave Trudee alone, so I told my friend I wouldn't be joining him. When Trudee heard that I would be staying home, she was adamant. "You've got to go!" she said. "My sister will come to take care of me and friends can fill in. You need time for yourself. Go for a week right after my time in the hospital. I'll be fine. I don't need you to hang around here. You'll have plenty of other chances to take care of me." I wavered, and then saw her point. Besides, I did want to go sailing. "OK," I said. "I'll call you every time we get ashore."

Trudee had had her cycle of chemotherapy without too much discomfort and was home. Her sister came. I went off for a week of sailing that I was sure would give me a chance to relax and renew my energy for the long winter that we both knew was coming. I flew to Annapolis, where my friend and his boat were waiting for me. As soon as I got off the plane, I called home. Everything was fine. "Have fun," Trudee said. Did I hear a catch in her voice? Or was it just my imagination? I met my friend and off we went. It was a relief to be on his boat. The taste of the salt spray, the sting of the fresh wind, and the motion of the boat itself all braced me like a tonic. There was no doubt about it: This was a good idea.

I called home that night, and Trudee sounded a little worse. Nothing too alarming, just the usual nausea and vomiting. She was in bed. Friends came to set up the stereo in our bedroom so that she could listen to music while she lay there. She wasn't interested in reading. "No, there is no reason for you to come home," she said. Each day she sounded worse than she did the day before.

In addition to my anxieties about Trudee, I had an obligation to stay with my friend. I had said that I would serve as crew, and he couldn't easily sail the boat without me. Having said that I would come along for the week, I was committed to staying through that time. More and more, however, my thoughts were with Trudee and not on the boat. In reality, I was not on that sailing trip after the first few days. I did the mechanical things I had to do, but all my emotional energy was with Trudee. Yet I couldn't get to her; I was trapped. By the time the week was up, I was an emotional wreck. I couldn't wait to get home.

When I saw Trudee, I was shocked at how pale and weak she looked. She lay in our bed, covered to the chin. A plate of uneaten food sat on the bedside table. A glass of ginger ale, with the ice mostly melted, stood beside it. The ever-present pink yerg bucket was on the floor next to the bed, and another smaller one was next to her pillow. Carefully, I gave Trudee a hug and a kiss. She smiled and said in a weak voice that she was glad I was home. "Not as glad as I am," I said.

Trudee recovered her strength as soon as she was taken off the high-dose ICE protocol. She never had another bout like that one. "I'll never do that again," I said to Trudee. In response, she always said the same thing: "Of course you will. You should have gone. And I'm glad you had a good time." I never argued with her, but I never agreed with her either. My absence was hard for her and even more difficult for me. I never forgot the feeling of being trapped where I should not have been. I never got over the feeling of catching fleeting reports of horrors and being totally helpless to do anything. I never forgot the pain of trying to be in two places at the same time: one, the concrete world of the boat and my friend, of chores and obligations, and of beautiful Maryland sunsets over the water that caused only anxiety and heartache; the other, a mental world that I tried to create from bits of what Trudee and her sister were telling me on the phone. From this picture I tried to judge whether I should just bolt to be with her. "Never again," I decided.

Establishing a New Normal Life in the Cancer World

All of which brings us back to the key question. "And how are *you* doing?" This is the question that summons us back to our painful reality. This is the question that crumbles our defenses, even though we need those defenses to get along, to maintain the façade of normalcy—even if it is a new kind of normalcy. And so we have difficulty answering the question. The more strongly we want to maintain the façade of normalcy, the more energetically we evade the question.

Naturally, we are ambivalent about the role we play as cancer partner. We want to be as helpful, supportive, loving, cheerful, strong, encouraging, and optimistic as possible. We want to be everything positive and life affirming for our partner. On the other hand, we see powerful threats to our own well being, happiness, and future. All those positive intentions do not jibe with the inevitable recognition of our own impotence in the face of the cancer experience. If we are lucky, things work out. If we are not lucky, there is little we can do to make them work out. We have to think about life in a different way.

Big changes are happening all around the cancer partnership, as well as within it. There are the obvious changes of our partner's health, strength, and attitude. There is the ever-present possibility of the biggest change of all—separation. There is our ambivalence about the shifting distance that is developing in the partnership and about the ultimate gulf that is looming, although the speed with which it is approaching is wholly unknown. There are new responsibilities that come with picking up the responsibilities that our partner has had to let go. Through all this, we cancer partners strive mightily to preserve a sense of normalcy for both partners.

What would make this cancer life more normal? More than anything we want someone else to go through the cancer experience with us. We try to stay as close as possible to our partner and to share that other view of life in the cancer world. But the sharing is always imperfect. We are left alone in one of the hardest and most complex roles we are ever to play in our lives. To a greater or lesser extent, we have lost the person closest to us. Even if the cancer treatment is going well, the preoccupations of the partner with the cancer are so different from those of the cancer partner that the experience is quite different for each of us.

Think of the cancer partners in their first weeks of living in the harsh beauty of the cancer world. They have pitched their tent out of the blistering sun that sapped their energy all day. They are weary from many days of walking, weighted by their terrible burdens. They curse their shoddy equipment, nothing like the light and elegant packs they had in their previous life on the other side of the border. Night falls and they rest, sleeping the fitful sleep of those who wander in strange places and are not quite sure of where they have decided to spend the night. The night sounds are unfamiliar. He wakes before she does, and in the early morning coolness, he gathers the sparse wildflowers to adorn the ridge of their otherwise bleak tent. She wakes, and seeing them, says, "I wonder how those weeds got stuck on our tent."

The cancer world is an emotional and intellectual world of our making. But there is a real world still out there. More than in that careless pre-cancer life, our hopes rise and fall on the basis on some new piece of information or feeling. This isn't exactly a fantasy world, but it is a world of hopes and fears that we construct for ourselves. As with everything else in the cancer world, however, the constructs are writ large. You cannot avoid them, and you cannot avoid recognizing them for the constructs that they are. Long-term survival in the cancer world requires direct approaches to the horror. Serious problems arise when we deny our own reality to ourselves. We partners can take vacations from time to time, back there across the border, and visit where we used to live. But for better or worse, the cancer world is our real home.

Anger and Other Rituals

A man said to the universe,
"Sir, I exist!"
"However," replied the universe,
"The fact has not created in me
A sense of obligation."
—*Stephen Crane,* **War Is Kind**

Despite all the intellectual sophistication and scientific insight we enjoy, our responses to sickness and the threat of separation and death are probably very much like those of our primitive ancestors who sat huddled in their cold, wet caves trying desperately to gain some control over what was happening to them. They painted human and animal figures and a variety of geometric shapes on the walls of their caves. They made small amulets and figurines to carry, and offered sacrifices of animals, people, and even things that they valued in hopes of striking a bargain with the forces that controlled life and death.

And us? Are we so different? We huddle in the caves of our cancer world and develop our own rituals for placating those same forces of death and destruction. We create our own amulets to ward off evil. Like our ancestors, we want to feel that our universe is not as impersonal and implacable as it appears. If it were, our suffering in the cancer world would be meaningless. The effort to make the cancer experience meaningful sometimes drives us to do things that would have been familiar to our prehistoric forebears.

On one of our first trips to the Dana-Farber Cancer Institute for Trudee's treatment, we met a friendly couple who was about a month ahead of us in the cancer life. We formed a quick friendship when, encouraged by his wife Rita, Al pulled up his shirt to show Trudee his new pheresis catheter ports; plastic tubes with small fittings on the ends came out of his chest. I remember feeling how *not strange* his gesture was, and how peculiar it was that it didn't seem strange. Trudee was about to have the same kind of central venous line inserted through her chest wall into a large vein. The point of this minor but invasive surgery was that the port would allow her to take chemotherapy conveniently without having the needle stuck in her immobilized arm for hours. Al extolled the virtues of his new ports. He and Rita were the first fellow travelers we met in the cancer world.

The next time we met Al and Rita was about two months later, in that same room at the Dana-Farber Cancer Institute. Trudee and I were waiting for the doctors to tell us the results of the CT scan she had after her first round of chemotherapy. We were anxious and frightened, but the presence of Al and Rita helped us pass the time. We were also feeling excitedly optimistic about the report we were about to hear. Based on our theory that Trudee's chemotherapy had to be rough to do the job well, and the rougher the treatment the more effective it would be, we were prepared to hear that Trudee's tumors had shrunk dramatically, or had even disappeared. We cautioned each other that total disappearance would be too much to hope for, and tried to be realistic. "Let this six-week course of treatment shrink them substantially," we said "and then another course or two will certainly get the cancer under control."

After what seemed a very long wait, we were called into one of the little examining rooms the doctors use for conferences with patients. They gave us the bad news with great compassion, but the news was still very hard to hear: After six weeks of the almost intolerable high-dose ICE protocol, Trudee's CT scan showed that the tumors had actually grown quite a bit. The big growth at the back of her abdomen—"retroperitoneal space," they called it—had grown, and the "nodes" in her liver had become more pronounced. The doctors had to take Trudee off high-dose ICE and start her on another treatment that might or might not work. No one could be sure. We knew only that the present treatment was not working.

I felt the walls of the examining room closing in on us and my vision became that sort of tunnel vision in which you become blind to everything peripheral. I riveted my eyes on the doctors' faces as they described where we might go from here. I was looking for a sign from them that *they* weren't desperate. They said that many options were open to us; it was just a matter of choosing one. They added that new possibilities were coming down the research pipeline. If we could buy time with one of the conventional treatments, they said, we would be in good shape when the new treatments became available.

Intellectually, we were having a meeting with the doctors about the pros and cons of various medical treatments. The microscopic structure of the tumor is such-and-such; the molecular structure of the chemotherapy agent is such-and-such; the empirical evidence regarding the clinical effectiveness of the treatment is such-and-such. The hard science was reassuring, but emotionally, we were talking about "buying time." That put us back in the cave, sitting on cold, damp boulders waiting for a sign from the painted figures on the stone walls that seemed to dance in the flickering light of the fire we built just below the stone outcropping. Should we kill a bear for its blood? Would a little black stone amulet bring us better luck? Should we sacrifice something? Someone? Should we try a six-week course of adriamycin? It was hard to tell one discussion from the other. Dreadful as that high-dose ICE protocol had been for Trudee, that treatment was now much more reassuring than the free fall we had just started. Suddenly, high-dose ICE was a familiar devil that was far more tolerable than the unknown devils that lay ahead.

We decided on a more conventional combination of chemotherapy drugs that had been somewhat effective in slowing the growth of leiomyosarcoma in some people. Three months passed. It was time for another CT scan and a review of Trudee's treatment. Trudee and I did the equivalent of scratching marks on smooth stones for whatever security they might give: Whenever we went downstairs to the CT scan room at the Dana-Farber Cancer Institute, I always sat in the same chair in the waiting room so that I could see Trudee go into and come out of the scan room. Every time, she would turn around just before she entered the scan room, smile, and flash me her thumbs-up, good luck sign. I would smile back and give her my own thumbs-up. Half an hour later, the door would open and Trudee would stride out, smile again, and we would repeat the thumbs-up. Did we really believe that this would bring good luck? Not really. Would it have been a serious breach of some unspoken contract between us if we neglected this private ritual of ours? Yes, most definitely.

This time, as we sat in the waiting room to be called into the little examining room for our report from the doctors, we were silent and terrified. Just as on the day of her previous CT scan report, Al and Rita were sitting there, awaiting their own appointment. We had not seen them since Trudee's last report, when they were sitting in the same waiting room. I was now shocked to see them. Their presence frightened me. In any other context, chatting with them would have been a pleasure for Trudee and me. That day, however, I felt that they were harbingers of bad luck. Their presence made me angry. "They have no right to ruin for a second time our chances of a good report," I thought. I felt that I needed to protect Trudee against malevolent forces that were represented by the coincidence of Al and Rita again sitting across from us in the waiting room. As luck would have it, Al and Rita were called for their own appointment with the doctor and we escaped sitting with them. I actually breathed a sigh of relief.

Living in the cancer world drives us back into deep, atavistic beliefs. Our friend Barbara told us about her family's Belgian good luck ritual of holding one's *duimekas*. You tuck your thumbs down into your fists, hold them up in front of you, and tell the person that you are holding your *duimekas* for him. At critical moments, Barbara would say that she was holding *both duimekas* for us. Did we think it would help? Not exactly, but it couldn't hurt. And as we wandered in the cancer world, the caves we found may have been uncomfortable, but at least they offered some shelter.

Another woman I met in the cancer world says that she watches the children outside her office window play basketball; if the kid makes the basket while she is thinking about her husband, it means that her husband will be all right. Another person uses traffic lights to predict her husband's future. If the traffic light stays green and she passes through the intersection without stopping, her husband's MRI that day will be a good one.

I spoke once with a person in the cancer world who himself is a physician. He is trained to be rigorously empirical in his approaches to the world. His own strategy for dealing with his wife's breast cancer is contrary to all his training and professional work. But he says it works. He does "little obsessive-compulsive things," he says, "because I feel like I have to do them." When he is getting undressed at the end of the day, for example, he puts his keys and his watch in their "special places" on his dresser. The keys always go in the basket, the watch never does. "I would not change these things because I have been doing them for a long time," he says. But he will "experiment" with newer things "to see how the patterns of what I do might change other things." When his wife's treatment was going badly and they were receiving only negative news, he thought, "Maybe if I change to tying my shoelaces left-handed, it will change our luck."

Another person, whose wife gets treated at a medical center in a city far from their home, does everything in exactly the same way on the days of his wife's treatments. When they go for treatment, they always stay in the same hotel. When they meet with their doctor, they always travel by the same route. They try to accompany the same people in the treatment program. "So far," he says, "this strategy has worked pretty well." This man, by the way, is a successful scientist. He is serious about calling this a "strategy," even though it is a "strategy" in the same sense that spitting three times before crossing water is a "strategy." But what is it a strategy for? Will tracing exactly the same route increase the effectiveness of his wife's treatment or change the data on the scan? Of course not. But it is a strategy for feeling less trapped by fear. It is a game many of us play to reassure ourselves that the universe is not implacable, that it notices what we do.

Demons jump out at us from their hiding places as we wander lost in the cancer world. As in a nightmare, apparently innocent gestures in the cancer world can provoke the most fearsome spirits. We could be walking along together, for example, enjoying the cool shade of a clump of trees on the arid plains of the cancer world. The little oasis might have a spring of cool water bubbling to the surface, and the clear water might run over pastel-colored rocks in a small stream that disappears into the bowels of the earth. Thinking that a cool drink would revive our partner's flagging energies and sinking mood, we might reach down and scoop some water for our partner to drink. We take the first sip, to be sure that the water is as sweet as it looks. It is. We offer the drinking cup to our partner, who gratefully accepts it and sips—and then vomits the water and the undigested lunch that was such a struggle to eat two hours earlier. The strategies we develop are our own ways of propitiating the spirits of that spring.

Many cancer partners carry or wear talismans to hold the cancer terrors at bay. One woman in the cancer world says that she is "not religious by nature," but that she always wears the St. Peregrine medal her sister gave her because St. Peregrine survived cancer. Another told me that once when she was driving, she stepped down hard on the gas pedal so that the hearse that was trying to pass her "wouldn't get ahead of me." She said she never did things like that before her husband got cancer. Another cancer partner, an academic, tells me that he himself doesn't carry a good luck charm, but says that he "probably should."

Soon after Trudee and I learned her diagnosis, she went by herself to tell her family about it. It was summer, so I stayed behind in our cottage on Sandy Neck, alone with my constant thoughts of Trudee. At that time, none of our friends knew what had happened. One night, as I sat on the front porch watching the green light on the buoy just off shore flash on and off, I decided to make a love knot for Trudee. We had been reading Annie Proulx's novel, *The Shipping News*, and because Trudee and I were both interested in sailing and the paraphernalia of sailing, we were intrigued by the knot metaphors in the novel. The love knot is a pair of interlocking overhand knots that a man at sea sends to his sweetheart back home. If she still loves him, she returns the love knot intact. If she is finished with him, she returns the knot untied.

I started first thing in the morning. I surprised myself at how much effort I put into making this knot. The elaborate, continuous pair of intertwined knots had to be just perfect. I tied and retied it until I was satisfied that the two loops were identical and that there were no twists in them.

Trudee loved the thing. When she went to the hospital for her chemotherapy or surgery, the love knot was the first thing we unpacked. I would hang it on the wall where Trudee could see it from her bed. That piece of rope assumed powerful meaning for us, and we would have been bereft had we lost it. The love knot was important, I think, not really because it would *give* us good luck, but because it was a tangible expression of our mutual *desire* for good luck. It obviously couldn't shape events in the real world, but it could help us shape our own anxieties about those events.

Memento Mori

When Trudee and I were in Costa Rica a few years before she got sick, we bought several small pieces of carved wooden folk art: a cow, a dog, and a skeletal figure that represented Death. All three figures were carved in the same primitive style. All had the same coloring: a white figure with large and crudely drawn anatomic details, and a vivid splash of red for the nose of the animals and the heart and pelvis of Death. The dog and cow looked naïve and playful. The memento mori looked like a child's fear carved into wood. The cow and the dog went into a corner of the living room. The skeleton went on a shelf in my study.

I would look at the memento mori from time to time, but after a while, I stopped seeing it. Time passed. A few years later, Trudee was diagnosed. More time passed. One day about a year after her diagnosis, Trudee said that the image of Death in our house was beginning to bother her. "Let's get rid of it," she said. I was shocked that I hadn't thought of this.

Getting rid of the figure turned out to be not so simple.

I am not a religious person. Nor would I call myself superstitious. I don't pray, and the idea that the universe can have any awareness of what it is doing to us is so alien to my nature that I could not be angry at what had happened to us. Yet the disposal of that memento mori became an unexpected problem. Why couldn't I just toss the thing in the garbage can? I didn't know why, but I couldn't. Once I realized that I couldn't take such a simple utilitarian course, disposal-with-meaning became a problem.

I thought of taking it out on the boat and tossing it overboard, but that approach was no good. First, I would never be out sailing alone. And for some reason, I wanted to be alone when I did it. More than one person necessarily made the event a ritual. The last thing I wanted to do was create (or worse, borrow) a ceremony for the disposal of a wooden figure we bought at a tourist shop in some dilapidated village in Costa Rica. Second, if I tossed the wooden figure overboard, it would likely float ashore somewhere. Worse, I thought it might float near the boat in full view but out of reach. Sure, I could attach weights to it and sink it to the bottom, but that, I thought, was getting a little too elaborate for my taste.

I decided to burn the memento mori in our fireplace. Burning it would solve the practical side of the disposal problem. And fire, that elemental force of nature, was a step toward dealing with the disposal-with-meaning problem, too. To do so, I had to wait until Trudee was away. I didn't want to do it with her around, and I certainly didn't want to do it with her. I didn't know why. I only knew that I felt delegated by Trudee to perform this little service for her. If she had wanted to, she could have thrown the figure in the garbage can as easily as I could have. Instead, she asked me to get rid of it for her. In retrospect, I see that this was one of those emotionally charged events in the cancer world for which life on the other side of the border hardly prepares us.

Trudee was away from home for a few days visiting her family. I was home alone. I wasn't planning anything until, almost without realizing it, without having made any decision but aware that I was acting out the conclusion to an inner argument, I was cutting kindling and laying it with great care in a star-shaped pattern in the fireplace. When the fire was ablaze, I laid the effigy of Death on top of the hottest part of the fire. A sentence formulated itself in my head as I went through the motions of committing the memento mori to the flames: "Death, I am not trying to cheat you or placate you, but I wish you could treat us more fairly." I repeated the sentence, mentally, as the flames began to char the paint. The legs went first because they were just spindly pieces of dry wood. The head fell off the body as the thin neck burned away. The ribs and red-painted heart and pelvis burned more slowly. Finally, the head caught fire.

I was very concerned that every bit of wood be consumed. I did not want Trudee to come home and find the head of Death resting among the ashes in our fireplace. I squatted before the fire, rooted to the spot until the whole figure had disappeared. The process took about half an hour. I was afraid that a telephone call or knock on the door would interrupt me at my ministrations. I was also afraid of what a friend might think if he came to the house while I was in the midst of my service. I had decided that I would not answer the doorbell if it rang. The whole thing would have been too difficult to explain.

When the fire burned itself out, I swept the ashes out of the hearth and scattered them on Trudee's flower garden. All the while I was thinking, 'I am going nuts. Am I going nuts?' I went back to my study and put a small gift Trudee had given me where the figure of Death had stood.

Superstition is a belief or practice that has its roots in ignorance, unreasoning fear of unknown or mysterious forces, or a false conception of causation. Magic is a superstitious rite in which ceremonies, charms, or spells are believed to have the power to cause a supernatural being to produce or prevent some event. Superstition made me fear the sight of Al and Rita in the waiting room. Magical thinking made Trudee and me continue the practice of the thumbs-up sign. I don't know what that spontaneous ritual of the memento mori was. In truth, it was almost a waking dream. Instead of mental events arising during sleep to express powerful emotions (if, in fact, this is what dreams do), this was a physical drama played out during waking time. Real fire destroyed real wood. Through it all, I reminded myself that I did not want to create a ritual; and of course, that is exactly what I did.

Anger

The roots of anger in the cancer world are very much like the roots of the ritual, superstition, and magic. The amulet works because we believe that something in the universe recognizes its power. This makes the cancer world a personal place. Whatever it was that insinuated us across the border, made our life hell. How could we not be angry at such an apparent assault? To make matters worse, having attacked us in such a brutal way, it then seems not to care. It is the carelessness of the attack that enrages us even more.

It is no mystery that being thrust into the cancer world makes us angry. "You never get a break," one cancer partner says. His wife had been through many hard times before her cancer, and then got the cancer on top of that. "Where's all the sunshine?" he asks. "Why?" He says that he gets "so damn frustrated and mad" because he sees his wife bitterly unhappy. "I just get angry at the situation, I get unhappy, and I hate the world."

We want to make the cancer life comprehensible. "You don't want your world to be without rhyme or reason," another cancer partner says. "You don't want to live in an irrational world." Her husband had a fast-growing form of esophageal cancer that is very rare in his age bracket. "It should not have happened to him," she says. Her husband didn't smoke or drink and was too young to develop that kind of cancer. They spent a great deal of money on organic foods. "Whatever we did, it wasn't good enough. And it makes me angry that there is no explanation. Things like this can't just happen to people."

Like the practices of magic, superstition, and ritual, anger assumes a universe that cares. It assumes a universe in which we can identify the source of the disaster. More than that, anger assumes that the source of the disaster is a personal one—a perpetrator—not simply a mechanism. Once identified as a force with a personality, we assume further that it can be placated and, if we are lucky, influenced to stop hurting us. We may call that force luck or God or fate. In any case, naming it relieves us of some of the burden.

But things like cancer *do* just happen. If I were a religious man, I would be angry. I think now of what a pleasure it would have been for Trudee and me to enjoy the luxury of growing old together. It didn't happen, and if I believed in a God, I would have a hard time accepting that his goodness could express itself in what happened to us. Instead, I sometimes think that I am the spiritual equivalent of colorblind. The words of faith just don't attach themselves to concepts or feelings for me. As far as I am concerned, our fates are what we make of the sum of accidents we call our life. Cancer happened when the little mistakes in Trudee's genes met with some poorly understood real-world events to let loose the dogs of cancer. In a universe like this, anger is a fiction we tell ourselves to make us feel better.

If you have been circling the block for twenty minutes looking for a parking place and you finally find one, only to have someone sneak into that space before you can back in, anger seems to be a perfectly reasonable response. You jump out of your car, shout at the guy, and hope to scare him or reason him out of your parking place. Failing that, you can threaten to escalate the encounter. How it ends is anybody's guess. Still, by raising your voice, vigorously moving your head and arms, and by adopting various threatening gestures, you hope (as the baboons and our other primate forebears do) to drive off the offending party. Sometimes it works. Other times the offending party drives us off. In either case, we probably feel better than if we had done nothing.

In a sense, our encounter with cancer is like the impotent rage we feel after the guy in the other car says he is not moving, his car is already halfway into the spot, and all you can do is retreat. Until you find another parking place, as you drive around and around the block, you may very well be aiming a few well-chosen words in his direction. But what does this fuming accomplish other than letting off steam? What if your partner is in the car at the time and you take your anger and frustration out on him? This corrosive anger can only lead from a bad situation to a worse one.

But what can we do when the world is what the problem is? If a downpour interrupts your picnic, can you honestly say that the weather made you angry? If your car stops running, can you get angry at the engine? If the roof of your house leaks, can you get angry at the shingles? The anger I understand has a real target that can *feel* and *appreciate* the force of my anger. We yell at the guy who pulls into our parking place. It's a bit more difficult to get mad at the universe.

A person I met in the cancer world says she is "furious" about her partner's cancer. She refuses to let the cancer be just an accident. "I don't know who else to blame but God, and I don't even know if I believe in God," she says. Another cancer partner says that right after her husband was diagnosed with a malignant brain tumor, she went down to the basement and took a big drink of whiskey. "I filled a water glass full and gulped it down like medicine." She got drunk fast. Lying on the floor, kicking her heels and pounding her head on the cellar floor, she felt that life was turning against her. She said that she had "a ball of anger that shot out into the world with no target and no ability to work it out." She remembered driving by herself, saying "Fuck you, God. I'm finished with you. You're a fucking bastard. Get out of my life." Eventually, powerless as she felt, she came to see the futility of her misplaced anger. Her husband would say, "Well, why not us? What would make us special that it wouldn't happen to us? Shit happens." She has come to agree with him, to some extent. "It isn't that I believe in a random or chaotic universe," she says, "but I don't believe that there's a universal ill will out to punish me either."

Trudee did say that the cancer made her very angry. She was not talking about herself only, but about the people in her support group, the people she heard about through the cancer grapevine, and about all the people with cancer who have to go through what she was enduring. "People have better things to do with their lives than to sit for hours having chemo dripped into their veins," she said. "People with otherwise busy lives are waiting in line to have their fingers stuck for routine blood tests. People who would rather be doing just about anything else are staring into their pink yerg buckets, waiting for the next wave of nausea." The waste and the indignity made her angry.

When Parallel Universes Collide

Trudee and I went to a night of comedy designed specifically to relieve the stress of living with serious illness. Not everyone in the audience was associated with the cancer life, but most of them were, judging by the number of head covers and wigs. It was an evening of jokes about how we make our lives miserable by assuming the worst of everything. We laughed heartily as the comedian transmuted the pain we knew so well into the absurdity of comedy.

The comedian's routines used a lot of props. After the performance, we discovered that copies of these props were on sale in the lobby. Trudee worked her way toward the table where funny faces, outlandish hats, and other things were on sale, at what I thought were outrageously high prices. "What do you want to buy?" Trudee asked. I really didn't want to buy anything. "Oh, just get whatever you would like. I'll be waiting over here," I said. I allowed the crowd to push me away from the table. In a short time, Trudee came back with a bright red, sponge rubber ball of a clown's nose. "How much was that?" I asked with an unmistakable edge in my voice. "Three fifty," Trudee told me, "Why?" We left, with Trudee wearing her new purchase.

I have thought about my testiness that evening. In absolute terms, the money was insignificant. But I was bothered by conflicting feelings. The sponge balls were certainly cheap enough for the presenters of that evening to have given them away. We would all have left with a bit of the good feelings that remained after a solid hour of laughing together. Selling the nose seemed to be an effort to exploit the suffering of the audience. I also felt trapped, in a way, into participating in this exploitation. If Trudee wanted to buy something, who was I to say no? We kept the red nose in the car. It was useful when we pulled up to toll booths or were stuck in traffic.

There are other times when the same drama gets played out, and the consequences are more significant. Trudee and I had heard about a Korean healer working in the Boston area who was having great success in combining his traditional healing methods with the conventional methods of modern medicine. We knew people who were drinking various teas or getting regular acupuncture or moxibustion treatments. We had no idea whether these treatment were having an actual therapeutic effect. But we did know that the people getting these treatments *thought* they were feeling better. I began to realize that if you *think* you are feeling better, you *are* feeling better. If these treatments could make Trudee feel better, why not?

I suspended my disbelief, and we went to the healer for a consultation. I remember feeling at the time that Trudee and I were splitting into parallel realities. A psychological reality was becoming more important than the physical reality. In the physical world, Trudee's tumors were leading lives of their own. We hoped that the chemotherapy would knock them down, but there was little we could do to influence events in the physical world of cancer. Instead, the *hope* that we might be able to do something effective became as important as the physical realities with which we lived. If going to this healer could affect this other dimension while the chemotherapy did what it was supposed to do, so much the better.

We went to his "clinic" in a sprawling, broken-down house in a poor part of town. We introduced ourselves to the receptionist and sat in the waiting area. To our left, a man and a woman were treating themselves by placing small bits of burning material on clearly marked spots of skin up and down their arms. The burning material filled the waiting area with a sweet smell of incense. Slowly and with a great sense of method, the man and woman worked their way up both their arms, igniting a small piece of this material in the flame of a gas lamp that sat on the table, and placing the burning incense on their skin. I watched them in silence as Trudee filled out a questionnaire about her general health and her specific complaint.

In a short time, Trudee and I were ushered into a large room where we met with the man himself. He wanted me to be present in the room during his interview and examination of Trudee. There was not much of an interview. He studied the questionnaire that Trudee had completed in the waiting area. Then came the physical examination, during which he felt her pulses on either side of her neck. "Ah," he said to me, "feel this." He invited me to feel Trudee's pulses, too. Taking my hands, he placed my thumbs on Trudee's right and left carotid arteries, as they went up her neck. My thumbs, I thought—I'm sure I'll be feeling my own pulse and not hers. Still, I did what he said. "Which side is stronger?" he asked. I answered, but apparently, I gave the wrong answer. He took my hands again and placed them on Trudee's neck, but this time he made sure that my right thumb was well away from her pulsing carotid artery on the left side of her neck. "Feel again. Which is stronger?" With a straight face, I answered, as he wanted, that her left side was weaker. Although I was getting furious at what I thought was his charlatanry, I didn't want to be too openly critical out of respect for Trudee's desire to believe in him.

"Your pulse is stronger on the right side because you have an obstruction of your energy on your left side," he declared. Trudee had described in her questionnaire the large tumor growing in her left retroperitoneal space. In the course of the examination, the healer told us nothing that he hadn't already learned from reading Trudee's answers on the questionnaire. He then attached three electrodes to Trudee's left arm. The first was at the level of her wrist, and the other two were at points higher up her arm. He plugged the leads into the electronic device that stood beside her chair and turned the dial. "This will show the energy flow to the lung, kidney, and liver." He pressed the button. He changed the setting of the dial. "And this will show the energy flow to the heart, spleen, and intestines." He pressed the button and printed the results on a strip of thermal paper.

The healer scrutinized the strip of printout and then asked Trudee her birthday. With this information, he consulted a book written in Korean. The page was ruled into several columns. He traced his finger down one of the columns, thought for a minute, and then rendered his conclusion. "You have a major energy blockage on your left side. I cannot help with this because you are taking chemotherapy." He did not suggest stopping chemotherapy. Nor did he suggest, as we had hoped when we first contacted him, combining traditional and conventional therapies. Trudee was visibly shaken, and I was upset for her. I was also getting impatient.

"I suggest you speak to my son," he said. He called for his son, who ushered us into another large room. He sat behind a large desk, and we sat in small chairs across the desk from him. Beside the desk was a very large bookcase filled with books. A few of the larger ones were in Korean. I was impressed. Then I realized that the other books were mostly cheap American paperback novels and five or six copies of the Boston University yearbook. The son launched a strenuous effort to sell us a host of products: vitamin supplements, blue-green algae, and a very expensive Korean tea. This part of the interview took about an hour.

I could see that Trudee wanted to come away from this visit with something tangible. She was very disappointed that the healer had refused to treat her. "I feel rejected," she said later, "and I failed acupuncture, too." At least, she thought, she could have some of the products that were being offered for sale. "I'll take a package of the blue-green algae. How much is it?" she asked. "Twenty-two dollars," he said. I cringed inside, but got myself under control, remembering my faith in the placebo effect. If she *feels* better, she *is* better, I reminded myself. "That's good," I said to her as reassuringly as I could. "Let's see how this works, and we can always buy more stuff later." Trudee was not listening. "I should probably take some of those other things, too," she said. Two hundred and fifty dollars later, we got into the car with a large bag full of teas, herbs, enzymes, algae, and food supplements.

I thought it was important for Trudee to feel that I was with her on this. Solidarity is key. Driving home, we talked about her disappointment and her skepticism about the whole process. I told her that I had a hard time believing what we heard but added, "What do I know?" When we had all the stuff we bought sitting on our dining room table, she asked me more pointedly, "Do you think this stuff can work?" "I doubt it," I said. "Yeah, let's take it back," she said. Which is what we did.

The point of this story is not whether the blue-green algae and the food supplements can work. As I said to Trudee, I really have no idea. The point of the story has to do with support. In this case, support was following Trudee wherever she wanted to go, suspending my own disbelief as long as she believed, and offering my own more critical view *when it was asked for*. Waiting to be asked was the hard part. If she had never asked me, I suppose we would have been stocking up on blue-green algae, enzymes, food supplements, and Korean tea every month.

Below the Anger

As we pass through the cancer world, we create many rituals to assure ourselves, first, that the universe notices our pain, and second, that acknowledging our pain imposes some obligation on the universe to treat us better. We desperately want relief from the terrible thought that our great pains can't be merely accidental. The same thinking that makes rituals so attractive—the belief that something in the universe is congenial enough to recognize our suffering—also sits within us as a pool of black anger. That pool of anger is fed by two main streams. One stream is the sense of being powerless. The second root is sadness.

Many people I met traveling in the cancer world said that they were angry at feeling powerless. Cancer had stolen their lives, they said, in various ways. It hurt them to see someone they loved going through unpleasant and painful things. They feared that they were soon going to lose their partner. They hated the thought that their own lives would be torn from them if they lost their partner. One cancer partner said to me that he "just wants to scream at some-body" because of "the unfairness of it all, the randomness of it all." If the doctors keep him and his wife waiting too long or if there is some kind of mix-up in the appointments, he gets very upset. He won't yell at his wife, he says, because "she did everything she could to avoid getting this cancer." He yells at the children, but then feels guilty about it. He yells at work. Coming back to work after getting bad news from the oncologist, for example, he has "a shorter fuse" than he usually does. "When people at work can see that it's been a bad day, they will leave me alone. But then that makes me angry, too. It kills me that nothing I can do will help the situation."

We might direct our anger at God. We may find ourselves alienated from the religion that once gave us succor in painful times. We may attack the person who is sick, the one who, we think, heaped all this trouble upon us. That is the cruelest feeling of all. "You can't be angry at a situation," one cancer partner says, "so I get angry at my hus-band." Then she gets mad at herself for attacking him. She says to her-self, 'What am I doing? The man has cancer. The fact that he is brain dead shouldn't bother me like that.'" There are angry moments or days when we can't do anything right to comfort the other person. There are times when we are repulsed by the physical care that is required. We may be angry at the medical system, the system on which we find ourselves so dependent. We may be angry at our fate. These are all things outside ourselves, as if that's where the problem resides.

In fact, although the cancer is outside us, the problem lives inside. The second root of our anger is sadness. One young mother said that she felt "robbed" of the enjoyment of being home with her children because of her husband's cancer. She feels "angry at the cancer" because "our lives have been clouded over." But then she rethought her explanation. "I mostly have been sad," she said. "Maybe I am angry that I am sad. I am angry at myself."

Our anger is how we try to protect ourselves against the sadness. It is a preemptive strike, perhaps to create a feeling that is just a little less uncomfortable than the sadness we don't want to feel. This kind of anger is black and brooding and not a jet of fire. We may say that we are raging against our fate, but in fact we are raging against our grief. There is nothing "wrong" with taking comfort in rituals or in anger. In fact, it says something about the human condition that we seek those ways of showing ourselves that the universe we inhabit is not careless and impersonal. Eventually, however, the anger and other rituals we devise get in the way of our finding the sadness that runs like small streams to a mighty lake in the cancer world.

The Double Life

Thus is man that great and true *Amphibium*, whose nature is disposed to live in divided and distinguished worlds.

—Sir Thomas Browne,
Religio Medici

The word "amphibian" means literally "living in both worlds" or "having a double existence." This perfectly describes the status of the cancer partner. Like a frog, which spends part of its life in water and part on land, the cancer partner lives in two worlds, but is never fully invested in either of them. One world is as solid as fear. The other is as tenuous as a wish. The world of fear is full of terrors too awful to consider. It is a world where quiet streams turn suddenly to torrents that sweep us onto submerged rocks we can hardly see. This is the cancer world that convinces us that we are helpless and that our situation is hopeless. In this world, even dangers that exist only in our fearful imagination throw us into that same vicious current.

At the same time, there is another cancer world where hope is cultivated. Here we plant the seeds of ease in fertile and well-watered fields. When those seeds finally germinate, we think, we will be safe once again, living in a world just like the quiet pre-cancer world we inhabited before crossing the border. The anticipated sweetness of that place seduces us into thinking that everything will work out fine. But we are also afraid to trust our hope. We cannot be sure that those seeds will germinate, and we are afraid that they cannot.

When Trudee and I married, we expected to enjoy a long future together. The marriage vow did include something about the possibility of death parting us, but that ultimate parting was so far in the future there was little point in thinking about it. When Trudee was diagnosed with leiomyosarcoma, our sense of time changed. The shock of that information forced us to live with a dramatically fore-shortened time horizon. We were not going to live "happily ever after"—that always was a fairy tale—but we still needed to live, even though our future could be blighted at any moment.

In our first understanding of what had happened to us, we knew that we might indeed have a future, but that it would be a horrible one. After living for a while with that sense of doom, and seeing that we were still getting along from day to day, putting one foot in front of another—almost like before—we saw the future more realistically. The feeling ripened in us gradually that we still had some kind of future, but we couldn't guess what shape it might take. Our amphibious life in the cancer world made agnostics of us. We were at home in two worlds; neither one was comfortable, but each was our natural element. Hope balanced fear precisely because we couldn't know the future.

It is an unstable balance, however. Trudee and I once went to hear Rosemary Clooney singing in concert. The music was familiar, the sound relaxing, the entire experience pleasant. Then, when Rose-mary sang the old chestnut "I'll be seeing you in all the old familiar places," Trudee and I suddenly choked up. We sat with tears stream-ing down our cheeks, feeling something too deep for words and so close to the surface that the song couldn't help but hit. The balance of hope and fear is easily tripped. In this case, but not always, fear had the greater weight, and we wept. The balance was so delicate, we found, that the slightest perturbation was enough to upset it.

The cancer partner's life is amphibian in another way, too. Most of us don't choose to avoid the cancer world completely, but prefer to shuttle back and forth between that world and the demands of the pre-cancer life. Work, friends, household obligations, and the sup-port—both practical and emotional—we need to give or arrange for our partners all take a great deal of our time and energy. Depending on how self-sufficient our partner is, we need to do more or less through the day to keep things going. Conflict between their needs and ours is inevitable. The doctor's appointment coincides with work obligations; staying home to provide care makes it impossible to buy the groceries; surgery must be scheduled for the holidays.

Conflicts like these are more than time conflicts. They are the con-trary pulls of two very different lives that can create discord between partners, even in the best of circumstances. Under the pressure of illness, anxiety, and dependency, the potential for trouble is great. We partners are not selfless saints. No one on either side of the border expects us to forsake our lives completely for the sake of our partners. On the other hand, many things need doing, and there are many things we *want* to do—things only we *can* do.

Hope on a Sliding Scale

Hope is really a sliding scale. "My wife has had chemotherapy and radiation for her breast cancer," says one cancer partner, "Although things are not great, I hope that they'll stay as they are. I don't expect things to get any better. But I am hoping that they don't get any worse." Some of us adjust our hopes as time goes on. "The doctor told us recently that we might have as long as ten years," one cancer partner told me. "That sounds like an eternity to me. Our hopes are on a shorter scale. With my partner's mental status so changed, I have to hope that I will be able to adapt quickly to the new life. I hope that we enjoy each other for whatever time we have. My hope is that she will live and that they will find a cure. My other hopes are to save enough money to get a house for us because it is important that she have a place of her own to die."

Trudee and I had to adjust our hopes to a new sense of future. The sight of a happy couple talking easily about the most commonplace events of their day or sitting beside each other at a concert or movie made me feel sorry for myself. It reminded me of all the things that were not to be for Trudee and me. I felt the burden of the great effort Trudee and I were making to maintain our sense of ordinariness in our increasingly extraordinary lives. Seeing the ease of others showed me how much we were losing. I envied those people in what Trudee and I called "the civilian world," people who were free of the intensity that we couldn't avoid in our cancer lives. Passionate intensity is a good thing from time to time, but as a way of life, it is excruciating. Trudee and I wondered aloud what happened to the days when the biggest decision was whether to go to a movie or stay home. What happened to the feeling that the future stretched out before us with no particular limit?

We got into the habit of planning for the short term. Plans to see a movie could be upset by some new symptoms or a sudden drop in

Trudee's energy. Planning a longer trip became an exercise in dealing with contingencies. We had to re-think our trips so that we would be near medical help if we needed it, where we could be sure that the blood supply was clean if she needed a transfusion, and where transportation was reliable if she needed to go to a hospital.

Living in the Present, Fearing the Future

Every summer, Trudee bought boxes of bulbs for fall planting. The tulips and daffodils would bloom the following spring with a careless profusion of energy that we more or less took for granted ("After all, a flower *is* a sexual organ," Trudee would say). It was very important to her that she order just the right assortment of bulbs, according to a theory of flower colors and shapes only she knew. Early in the fall, she would drive out into the country to pick up the stock of new bulbs she had ordered.

The summer of Trudee's diagnosis was no different from our previous ones. The month after learning her diagnosis, she spent days poring over the catalogs and bought her stock. This time, however, when fall came, the bulbs sat neglected in their boxes on the porch. We were both too frightened and exhausted to cultivate life in the harsh new world we had entered. The soil in the cancer world seemed far too flinty to nourish flower bulbs. We were afraid to project ourselves into a real future by planting those bulbs that would lie dormant until the following spring. The effort to build a new life out of the rubble that remained available to us was too painful. To play at planting tulips and daffodils was like burying the seeds of our own emotional destruction. We feared the future. Why should we decorate it with flowers of hope? The boxes of bulbs sat on the porch, mute tokens of the easy optimism we used to share.

The cold New England winter was approaching. Trudee's first experimental treatment protocol (a treatment the doctors called high-dose ICE) had its predictable and undesirable effects on her strength, appetite, and sense of well being. We did very little beyond our struggle to get through the day. Finally, as winter was almost upon us, Trudee and I both realized that if we waited any longer to plant the bulbs, the ground would be too frozen to dig and the bulbs would freeze to mush in their boxes on the porch. All Trudee's efforts that previous summer would have been for nothing. One Saturday afternoon she said, "Well, I don't know if I'll even see them come up in the spring, but I think we ought to plant those bulbs."

I hastily got out the dibble to poke small holes in the ground and the power auger to drill the larger holes, and we went to work. The season was already turning foul. It was getting late in the day, and Trudee's energy would last only so long. I made the holes, and Trudee, half sitting, half lying on the freezing ground, put the bulbs in the holes along with a little fertilizer and a shake of cayenne pepper to discourage the squirrels. I put the cold earth back over the bulbs and stepped the dirt down. We planted all the bulbs in one urgent session.

There is a kind of denial, if that is the right word, that makes it possible to fight *for* life while ignoring, as much as possible, all the things it would be fruitless to fight *against*. We never minimized the threat of Trudee's illness from ourselves or from other people. We simply chose to focus on other aspects of Trudee's condition. To deny what the disease can do and to forego potentially successful therapy is foolish and self-destructive. The kind of denial that says everything is fine when it is not is lying to yourself. You can't live your life sitting around expecting death. It is an effort to hold fast to what is positive and not to be undone by the fear of terrible things that might happen.

The fact that winter came and went and that we did both see the bulbs come to life the following spring is less important to me now than the fact that we planted them at all. Winter stood between our painful present and an uncertain future. Spring was what we were fighting for. For people who feel cut off from their future, living becomes meaningless. As long as we could feel that we still had a future, we could believe that our immediate lives were relatively normal.

All too soon, we came to live with an even more drastically foreshortened future. Eventually, a hospital bed was set up in our living room. A long plastic tube stretched across the rug, from the large oxygen tank in the corner to where Trudee sat propped up by five or six pillows. She needed supplemental oxygen all the time and had great difficulty moving her swollen legs. Her feet were up on a hassock, with two soft foam wedges to support her legs. I did what I could to make her comfortable by placing, moving, and replacing the pillows around her. When the pillows were finally in just the right places, we could both relax, satisfied for a time. Eventually, our time span contracted to those moments when there was no pain. The past was irrelevant. A new pain would soon erupt or Trudee would want to move from the chair to the bed or to the bathroom. That reset the clock, establishing a new present. The immediate past, that moment of respite, was already irrelevant ancient history. The best we could hope for was another moment of relief.

It is hard to describe the mutual tenderness of those times. We both knew that our future was reduced to the smallest possible increments. Yet normal time went on for people around us. The visiting nurse might call to say that she would arrive a few hours late because she had a meeting at her daughter's school. But we were living in a world of our own time in which clocks and calendars were useless. Medications that once were dispensed on a regular schedule, twice a day or every four hours, now were taken as needed.

Meanwhile, time became my regular preoccupation in other ways, too. Whenever Trudee drank something or peed, I measured the amount and recorded the time and volume in a little notebook. These numbers and her weight, which we also measured every day, fueled our daily hopes and disappointments. More urine was good; less weight was good. The simple numbers in my notebook, dutifully recorded with the time and date, summarized a host of physiologic processes and emotions as the passage of time signaled our approaching fate.

Then I was shocked to realize that our past was in jeopardy, too. Trudee's study had always been a mess. She liked that piles of papers, books, clothes, old cameras, catalogs, photographs, pieces of junk, and an assortment of belongings got parked there. So it was startling to see her sitting on the floor of her study one day, surrounded by large trash bags, sorting through her stuff. When I asked her what she was doing, she said that she was cleaning out her study. The way she said it, however, I thought she said *clearing* it out.

I had an idea that she wanted to have her files in good order before the time came when she would no longer be able to do it. I also thought she might be straightening out the memorabilia of her life. Working with her memorabilia, I thought, was her effort to edit her past before I became its conservator. A great wave of sadness came over me, and I went back downstairs, leaving her to her work.

Sometime later, when Trudee was away visiting her family and I was home alone for a few days, I thought, "So, this is what it will be like without her. This is a rehearsal for when she is dead." I could already feel the emptiness of the house and the reality of my loneliness. Ordinarily, I liked being alone some of the time. But this feeling was different from that relaxing and self-sufficient sense of myself. This was a painful anticipation of a time when Trudee would go away and not come back. I feared it would be a time when I would be locked in the painful present, a stasis that would never open to what is about to happen. The telephone would never ring. I would be cut off from everyone. I would wallow in the grief of having lost Trudee, having lost the life we enjoyed, having lost the future. In this circle of hell within the cancer world, nothing would happen.

Hopes and Gains

Before we crossed into the cancer world, the life of our partnership was marked by gains of all kinds and the hope of gains. The acquisition of *things* was the simplest kind of gain, but not the only kind. Trudee and I bought a house, planted bulbs that increased visibly from year to year, bought a pot or a chair if we needed one. The objects themselves were fun to buy, but the more important gain was the life we were building. Things were the scaffolding that supported our life. Still, things are only things. We expected the store of experiences we would have together to be our greatest gain.

After we crossed into the cancer world, all we could see ahead of us were the losses. Anyone who has entered the cancer world knows that wherever you look along the highways of that inhospitable world, there are scraggly processions of refugees marching alongside the road, carrying their present necessities and family treasures. Their progress is painfully slow, at times, because of the great burdens slung over their backs or pushed before them in crude carts. People who are too weak to walk sit by the roadside, holding photographs in large wooden frames of themselves and of their families. Others, thinking that gasoline will be available just around the next bend in the road, push their cars for as long as they can before abandoning them forever. Most of the people realize that they cannot continue like this for long and abandon the photographs, the family silver, the jewelry, the cars, the diaries and letters. These things are free for the taking at the side of the road. A few people stop to pick up something that catches their eye, but in a short while they learn to ignore the discarded treasures, too. Freed of that burden, they carry only their present.

Living in the two worlds of hope and fear makes buying things or giving gifts a problem in the cancer world because it sends tendrils of hope into an uncertain future. The first winter of our cancer life, for instance, Trudee refused to buy a much-needed winter coat. Her old one was nothing but the inside and outside nylon layers. All the down that once filled the space between had broken down, leaked out, or resettled at the bottom of the coat. She was always cold. We were warned that chemotherapy would sap her energy and make it even harder for her to stay warm. Still she resisted buying a coat. Trudee had her reasons for not buying one: "This one will do fine for now." "Coats are so expensive." "Maybe I can borrow a coat from somebody." Finally, I had to bully her into seeing the absurdity of what she was saying. All the time, however, I was realizing how painful these diversionary tactics were, for her and for me. Trudee was really saying, and she knew it, that it might not be worth spending the few hundred dollars on her for a new coat because she might not be around long enough to warrant the expense.

Buying presents for each other was an even more delicate matter. In our pre-cancer life, the presents we bought each other were sometimes tied to conventional occasions like birthdays or anniversaries, and sometimes they were just gratuitous acts driven by bargains, happenstance, or love. Giving presents was different in our cancer life, but it took me a while to recognize the difference. Trudee bought me several fairly expensive gifts. When I tried to talk her out of getting them for me, she said that these were things to remember her by. She wanted me to have physical things that would continue to exist after her.

From me, however, she wanted something quite different. She wanted emotional things that would vitalize the moment. Over the years, for instance, I would make her very elaborate cards from pictures I cut out of magazines and pasted on a long roll of paper with goofy text. That's what Trudee wanted me to give her. She didn't want things that had more of a future than she had. She wanted only things that had their presence rooted deeply in our past, but that lived in the present.

Losses and Fears

Although we live our amphibian existence in two worlds, we always carry something of the one world into the other. A cancer partner I met traveled to England, Scotland, and Wales with his wife about a month after an operation on her breast and the removal of a piece of her rib for a biopsy. The doctor told them that they had "a narrow window of time" before the start of chemotherapy, so they left home with high hopes.

About four days into the trip, his wife developed such a sharp pain in her hip that she couldn't walk. Her hip had bothered her occasionally at home, but there was no obvious cause of her pain. The doctors didn't think her pain was anything serious. But once they got to London, the pain became intolerable, and she couldn't walk. She stayed in the hotel room while he explored the city on his own. He brought meals back for the two of them to share. "This was a very sad time for me because I could see what was coming in our lives," he says. The rest of the trip they spent in the car. Still, he was "haunted by the feeling that something was changing. I felt that we were being stalked by something I didn't know and didn't like." When they got home a month later, they learned that his wife was a developing a metastatic tumor in her hip.

Trudee and I marked a similar loss on a trip to New Mexico about a year and a half after her diagnosis. She had been in chemotherapy for more than a year. The day was one of those clear, hot, dry days that amazes Easterners like us, when the vanishing point of earth and sky seems to be at an infinite distance. We remarked on how understandable it was that people living in a place like this would develop a mystical bond with the land. In fact, while we were there the genius of the place affected us, too.

We wanted to explore the ancient cave dwellings at Puye, just outside Santa Fe. As we drove into the small parking area at Puye, two routes lay in front of us. One route was straight ahead: a series of crude log ladders that scaled the cliff from one terrace to the next. A second route was the access road that we could drive to the top of the cliff. For a long moment, we considered the two options. We both anticipated the joyful struggle we would face in climbing those ladders to the top of the cliff. We had driven for more than an hour, so the prospect of clambering up the face of the cliff was a pleasant one. But, of course, we had forgotten the third member of our party, the cancer and the residual effects of Trudee's recent chemotherapy. "You can climb and I'll wait here," she said. I knew that wouldn't feel right. With an unpleasant shock of recognition that our former impulses were no longer appropriate, we sat in the car studying the ladders and imagining ourselves climbing to the top. Then I restarted the car and drove up the dusty road that skirted the cliffs and brought us to the top.

Once at the top of the cliff, we clambered down the few narrow steps that the Indians had cut into the rock face to the topmost terrace of the cliff dwellings. Trudee had a very hard time climbing down. The transfusion of red blood cells she had had before we left on this trip had given her enough energy for normal activities, but not for the combination of physical exertion and high altitude. Her legs were trembling and cramping; she was terribly short of breath. I was afraid that she wouldn't be able to climb back up the steps if she continued to over-exert herself in exploring that first terrace. So, with me climbing behind her and literally pushing her up the stairway, we struggled back to the top, where Trudee collapsed on a rock. Without a hint of self-pity, she insisted that I go back down to the caves and explore them for the two of us.

My return to the terrace was filled with complicated feelings. I knew that Trudee was safe and comfortable so there was no need to worry about her physical well-being. But I carried with me her regret at not being able to share this little adventure as we had done so many times in the past. I felt sorry for Trudee; I felt sorry for myself for being deprived of her. I also felt a responsibility that enriched the moment for me by requiring that I live it for the two of us. "Tell me what you see," Trudee called out as I descended the stone steps. I took the mission seriously and looked with greater care so that I would have interesting things to report when I got back. These threatening losses remind us that worse is coming. We can be thankful for what has remained, but the remnants of those familiar things now lost make us fear what more there is to lose.

Other losses are more absolute. Important things go without any hope of their return. The stresses of illness and the illness itself can so change a person with cancer that we partners may wonder how that could be the person we fell in love with. Just as the cancer grows as a physical intruder in the body of the partner, so changes in attitude, outlook, and personality can make the other person seem a stranger.

One cancer partner says it already feels as if she has lost her husband. Before his illness he was confident and gregarious, happy and fun. His cancer made him an angry and frustrated man. "He is not as trusting of the world, not as trusting of his own strength, and he is not as trusting of me. It's like being with a different person." She says that in the course of all these changes, she lost a part of herself as well. "I have had to learn to accept my loneliness. I have lost that secure feeling that I could depend on other people. Now I feel that I am the only person I can rely on."

Another cancer partner says that she can't share anything about herself with her husband. "Our relationship is so altered by the tumors in his brain and by what the radiation treatment has done to him that he wouldn't get it," she says. She has had to accept that her husband is no longer autonomous and never will be. The transition from being a functioning and thinking man to a completely dependent person has been hard for her.

Intimacy can go, too. Physical love in the cancer world is possible, but it is not the same as in the pre-cancer world. People who are sick, worried, tired, uncomfortable, and in pain are in no mood for making love. Partners may be put off by physical or emotional changes they see in the other person and may feel distant.

The disease or the treatment can make the mechanics of physical love impossible. One cancer partner says that she and her husband have known each other for more than forty years. "So many things are gone since my husband got prostate cancer," she says. They have lost their financial security, their work, the feeling that they will live happily ever after, and the feeling that they will retire and grow old together. Because of his prostate cancer, they have also lost sex totally. "That is a great loss for both of us," she says. "As wonderful as it is to have my husband still alive, and as intimate as we can still be in our lives together, I don't feel as close to him physically now that we no longer have sex. I miss the physical love we used to have. That is not replaceable." This is a big issue for them because whenever they talk about it, he gets upset and angry. Then her husband becomes overwhelmingly sad. "His sadness seems to me to be too great a price to pay for my own satisfaction, so I don't push."

Bad Thoughts

Either way, in the cancer world, we have very troubling bad thoughts. "When I first thought about my wife's funeral early in this process," says one cancer partner, "it was a horrifying thought. It felt disloyal, even sadistic, to be planning for the event that I fear the most." In the double life we lead, thoughts of the worst that can happen are painful and inescapable. But so are thoughts about the best that can happen. We naturally fear the worst, and are afraid to hope for the best.

The cancer world is no different. We visit certain places in that terrain at our peril. There is the Grotto of our Partner's Death, the Forest of Our Loneliness, the Desert of What Is to Come, the Maelstrom of Despair. If we can see these places from a distance, we sometimes can avoid them. Other times, we are suddenly in the grip of the spirit of one of these places. Sometimes we deliberately put ourselves in one of these frightening grottoes or chasms to see what it feels like. Regardless, on our trek through the cancer world, we will visit the places of bad thoughts. These troublesome thoughts are ways of dealing emotionally with this potentially catastrophic situation. The kinds of thoughts that come to us—wishing the spouse dead, planning to get married afterwards—are normal. The hardest part is allowing those painful and frightening emotions to come up.

The mind is always engaged, even when we think it is idling in neutral. "One trembles to think of that mysterious thing in the soul," Herman Melville writes in *Moby Dick*, "which seems to acknowledge no human jurisdiction, but in spite of the individual's own innocent self, will still dream horrid dreams, and murmur unmentionable thoughts." Down in the secret places of the mind that spawn the night dreams and the day thoughts that we try so hard to drive back into their hiding places, another part of the mind is coming up with its own notions of what it is like to be the cancer partner. The things furnished by that other mind can be quite frightening. We can be horrified to realize that we are capable of some of these feelings and thoughts. It would be a mistake, however, to dismiss these outcroppings of raw emotion as merely "irrational" or "impulsive" or "hysterical." They are as much "us" as the noble thoughts we also are capable of inventing.

Probably the worst "bad thought" is the one about the death of our partner; and it comes anywhere, unannounced. "When I filled out the income tax form this year," one cancer partner says, "I wondered whether this might be the last year that we would be filing jointly as a married couple. I had thoughts about how it would be easier for me if she died. These thoughts trouble me because what's happening is evil. I try to get out of that mood as soon as I can. I believe it is detrimental to have those thoughts."

Says another cancer partner: "When I was first dealing with my husband's cancer, I already had him dead. I knew he wanted to be cremated, and I planned how I was going to do it. I started to think about where I would put the urn with his ashes. I thought about what it would be like to get on with my life without him. I am alone, and his distancing himself from my own pain is making me angry. If we're waiting for something to die, what will it be—my husband or the relationship? We may never get back together again, and that makes me sad. Then I feel guilty for even thinking this way."

Another cancer partner talks about the "enormous guilt" associated with his mixed feelings about his wife's eventual death. Although he recognizes that "there is likely to be an ending to the pain some time in the future," he says, "it kills me to think that my wife has to die to give me the relief that I want. That is a thought that I cannot let go of." For him, the worst thing that could happen is painfully mixed with his hope for eventually having an easier life for himself.

Another cancer partner is bothered by what she calls her "many unsayable things." Her most awful thought was that "there would come a time when I would want my husband to die. The easier his death and the sooner, the better, as far as I was concerned." She was hoping that he would get better, but she also *knew* that his untreatable cancer would almost certainly progress. "You are never completely rid of the shadow and the sense that an anvil is hanging just overhead. It was a terrible feeling to have. I would say every so often that I just wanted to put the burden down for a while." When her husband was first diagnosed with esophageal cancer, she said she was "mentally fast-forwarding." At some point—one year? five years? twelve years?—he would no longer be here. It was terrifying for her to think about trying to pick up her life and start over. "For some bizarre reason, it was even more terrifying to think about limping along for twelve years, with my husband in and out of hospitalizations. My life would be held in abeyance or thrown aside, and the next decade of my life would be devoted to his illness." She hated to think that way, and would force herself to put aside those thoughts. "Then other thoughts would creep in. The whole time I felt as if my being was fragmenting into multiple personalities."

We can think of these outcroppings of bad thoughts as hypothesis testing. Anyone who has tried to solve a hard problem knows the experience of having solutions pop spontaneously into mind, sometimes at the strangest times. Most of these "solutions" turn out to be illusory. Occasionally, however, a real solution comes to mind and the problem is solved. So it is with the vast emotional problem of living as a cancer partner. The mind presents possible "solutions" to that thorny problem. Most of the proposals are no solutions at all. Precisely because they aren't solutions, and because in reality there is no adequate solution, the mind keeps trying.

I had plenty of bad thoughts, myself. There were times when the whole thing felt too much. The overload was usually a pile-up of small things that needing doing just at the time Trudee needed me for something. The dog always seemed to want to go out when Trudee needed lunch or a drink of juice. Work often refused to be nudged aside when Trudee had to go to a doctor's appointment. I could miss a routine event like a scheduled blood test. After a while, even transfusions became familiar enough for Trudee to go alone or with a friend. But doctors appointments were inviolable times to be done together. I suppose I felt I was giving Trudee support. But I went with her to these appointments—our appointments is how I thought of them—as much for myself as for Trudee. I wanted to hear how we were doing, especially if the news was good. If the news was bad, I certainly wanted to be there to soften the blow, if I could. Those trips to get the results were always difficult for us. The day-to-day activity of going through treatment was unpleasant, but it was done in hopes of getting us something. It kept us busy. The day of the CT scan was the reckoning of whether the treatment got us anything or just kept us busy.

Almost from the day of Trudee's diagnosis, it seemed to me that wherever we drove, the roads were filled with hearses. I remember driving along the highway with Trudee one day a few months after she was diagnosed, and passing a long car transport trailer with four shiny new hearses aboard. We literally averted our eyes as we passed, and I noticed that neither of us commented on the unusual sight of four hearses stacked on a trailer. In other times, we certainly would have. When we drove past a cemetery, too, our otherwise animated conversation would catch its breath and falter. I knew that Trudee was thinking about those people already in their graves and wondering what it was like for them to get there. She was wondering about what her own dying would be like. Although she and I talked about almost everything, we never touched the subject in this way.

Once we were driving back from Trudee's treatment at the Dana-Farber Cancer Institute, and a small bird fluttered in front of our car. I am not sure what happened next. I think the car hit the bird and knocked it to the pavement. It happened so quickly, and the whole event was so odd and unexpected, I thought I might have imagined it. I remembered that soon after Trudee was diagnosed, she noticed a sparrow sitting on a branch on the shrub right next to our front door. The bird didn't fly away when we walked out the door; in fact, we could walk right up to it. When we did, it was obvious that the bird was sick. Trudee insisted on bundling the bird in a box and taking it to a vet for treatment. I got a small box, lined it with rags, and placed the sick bird in the box. Trudee drove off with it. She came back about half an hour later, in tears. The bird had died on the way to the vet, and Trudee had buried it at the roadside. Many months later, when this other bird fell (or seemed to have fallen) in front of our car, I was so shaken by what might have happened that I couldn't ask Trudee if she had seen it too. In my volatile emotional state, it seemed as if these little messengers of death were bringing their frequent reminders. Rather, these were the screens onto which I projected my own worst thoughts.

The thought did cross my mind more than once while driving along the highway or on the short drive back home from the Dana-Farber Cancer Institute that our problems would be solved so neatly if I just turned the steering wheel slightly to the right and ran into a wall. Other times I thought of the stash of drugs Trudee had accumulated through the years of her treatment. She had enough pain-killers and sleeping pills to put us both away. I think it was the French writer Albert Camus who said that the *possibility* of suicide was what kept him alive. He knew that he had a choice. The horde of pills gave Trudee security. She believed that as long as she *could* do it, she wouldn't need to.

I worried about what I would do if Trudee were in intractable pain, with little hope of improving her underlying condition, and she then turned to her horde of pills. How could I allow her to take her own life without also taking my own? The thought surprised me when it appeared; and I thought about it quite seriously. Trudee and I might have talked about it in a vague and hypothetical way, but it was never a plan. It was one of the many hypothetical solutions to a problem that existed more in my fears than in reality.

The Double Nature of Hope

In the cancer world, we hope with one side of our mind, and then we pull the hope back with the other. Hope says, "It could be." Experience says, "Unlikely."

"My hope today is very fragile," a cancer partner whose husband was not doing well told me. "I say that I hope certain things will happen, but I don't really believe it. I am really afraid that those things are not going to happen. My only strong hope is that his treatment, because it was so experimental and so toxic, will hold his cancer in place indefinitely. But I don't have any real hope that a new treatment will cure his cancer. The new treatments in development now may give a man another few more months. That doesn't sound like hope to me. My hope would be that it doesn't come back at all; but that is an impossible thing to hope for."

By the time Trudee and I got to the surgery option, we were well acquainted with the double nature of hope. We had been living with the cancer for a few years. In those years, it wasn't the realized fears, but rather the dashing hopes that broke our hearts. Some of the things we hoped for did happen. The cocktail of chemotherapy drugs Trudee got did shrink her tumors somewhat. That partial success gave us reason to believe that other things could succeed, too. We clung to the hope that drugs just over the horizon, still in the early trial stages, would turn out to be effective against Trudee's particular form of leiomyosarcoma. It was a race of research against the cancer. History was on the side of the cancer. So far, the disease always won the race. At least, we thought, the current cocktail would maintain the status quo. Then the standard treatment cocktail stopped working. Research was not coming up with much to support our hopes. Surgery became our only hope. We were told that surgery was a long shot, but not impossibly long.

Hope is contrary to experience by definition. This is what makes it so difficult. The evidence says one thing, hope says another. We want to believe in the better outcome, so we choose hope and minimize everything our experience tells us to the contrary. We hope that this time things will be different. Sometimes they are. This is like Pascal's wager that it is a better bet to act as if you believe in God than to lead a strictly atheistic life because, if God does not exist you gain nothing but lose little, and if God does exist, you gain much and would have lost more. This is even more true of hope in the cancer world. If events prove the hopes false, you have not lost much and have gained something by living hopefully. If, however, events can sustain the hope, you have gained a great deal and would have lost even more had you suffered in the clutches of hopelessness.

Without hope, there is no reason to go through all the discomfort, pain, tedium, anxiety, and effort of treatment, follow-up, testing, and more treatment. Without hope, there is really no reason for getting up in the morning. A lot has been written on the benefits of keeping a positive attitude. That may or may not be true, but it is obvious that the opposite is certainly true. A great deal of research on animals and people shows that hopelessness can kill. People who give up die sooner than those who keep up the belief that there is something to live for.

A cancer partner described living with her husband's illness as "a walk down a long staircase. Some piece of bad news tumbles you down the stairs, and you rest for a long time on the landing. Then with some new development, you suddenly head down another flight of steps until you reach a new landing. The new landing is a welcome resting place until another catastrophe comes to knock you down to a lower landing."

When we are living with progressive cancer and dealing with its treatment, the downward course feels inevitable. The "landings" are welcome respites along the way. What she didn't capture in that image was the description of the staircase itself. It would be an interesting exercise, indeed, to try to draw that staircase. For some people, I am sure, it would be a closed in, grim staircase, like the concrete and windowless fire stairs in a public building. Bare light bulbs in wire cages give a dim light to this strictly utilitarian descent. For others, however, the staircase could be a beautiful creation, with gracefully turned mahogany balusters, curving from one landing to the next. Large windows above can let sunlight onto the stairway during the day and a glimpse of the moon at night. On such a staircase, resting on the landings can be wonderful.

The realistic part is in understanding what are legitimate hopes and what are not. We could *wish* for a miraculous cure. That would be unrealistic. We could *hope* for the chance to make good use of the time we happened to get. I was walking in the parking garage of the Dana-Farber Cancer Institute when I overheard a conversation between two men. "You look great," one man said to the other. "How have you been doing?" "Well, I've been cancer-free now for almost six years." There was a short pause, and then the first man said, "May you live another day."

The middle ground is the difficult part of hope. The other person looks to the partner for an indication of how things are going. As a result, we are obliged to put a good face on, even while acknowledging that the situation may be serious. This can make it difficult for us partners. One woman had to go to the garage to cry because if her husband saw her tear-streaked face, he would assume that she was crying because, as he said, "she didn't think he was going to make it."

Hope also brings fears of its own: the fear of disappointment. When Trudee was going through her first chemotherapy, we expected the high-dose ICE protocol to shrink her tumors and, if not cure her, at the very least give her "a good long time." We never defined what that "long time" might mean. We just expected that the treatment would be effective. When it didn't shrink the tumors, and in fact allowed them to grow larger, we were not disappointed. We were terrified, but not disappointed. I think *disappointment* logically follows *hope*. Our thinking at that time was entirely different from that. We expected a positive outcome and then had to deal with the terror of recognizing that our thinking was just plain wrong. We were too sure of ourselves to hope. In time, however, we had to scale our thinking down from expectation to hope. "I am afraid to hope," Trudee said to me as we drove to New York for the consultation with her surgeon.

Hope depends on the imagination. Today we use the word "imagination" much more loosely than they did in the past. Not too long ago, "imagination" was a technical term meaning, among other things, the ability to divorce yourself from the concrete data of the senses in order to create something new. It also had a psychological dimension, in that time before psychology was invented. Imagination was the faculty that allowed us to get inside the lives of other people. Without this empathy, the role of the partner is reduced to doing chores. With it, the chores are transformed to loving and meaningful acts of devotion.

On the other hand, since the imagination is a move away from the evidence of the senses, there is always the danger that it is not to be trusted. The imagination can get you into a lot of trouble by conjuring up the worst fears and making them seem all too real. There is also the danger of thinking you understand what is going on inside the other person, when all the time it is the projection of your own anxieties and fears and hopes onto the other person. The best antidote for this error is checking with each other.

Someone once said that we should live life as if it were a comedy, knowing all along that it is a tragedy. The cancer makes us welcome even the most conditional resolutions of those complications. The role of the partner is to provide as many of those provisory defeats of the complications as possible, to keep up the saving illusion that life can still be a comedy. That is where the gallantry is found, and the generosity of the partner is in doing this for both. Comedy cheats these complications.

Trudee and I rented "My Cousin Vinnie" and laughed all the way to the end, and then we started to cry. Other comedies had the same effect on us. Why do we cry at the end of comedies? I think it is because the comedy is over. The comedy was exactly the opposite of what we were going through. In the comedy, we took great pleasure in seeing the characters tie themselves into knots, with the real world conspiring, it would seem, to pull the knots tighter. Since it is a comedy, we know we are in for a happy ending. By the end of the movie, the complications will all prove superficial and the loving couple will fall into a hug that says to us that all is right with the world. All difficulties resolve.

The hard part, however, is to do it in such a way that you both don't actually fall for the illusion. Honesty does require, after all, that you realize that you are doing the best you can, but that you can't really cheat reality. Que será será. What will be, will be. A story will be played out, and it will be played out beyond our or anyone else's control. This is always true. Even in the pre-cancer civilian life, most of what we do is out of our complete control. Nevertheless, we go on with our lives as if we had control. The trick of living in the cancer world is to keep up that attitude, even though the cancer has finally pricked the illusion.

The Singular Life

Nearly everything in the cancer life forces us into a double life. We live simultaneously in hope and fear, future and present, wish and reality, health and cancer, the other person's life and ours. For us to survive in the cancer world, however, we need to resolve these opposed pulls as much as we can. We must try to make a singular life where all we can see are dualities. The surprising thing is that the cancer can actually help us do this.

Trudee was in the throes of chemotherapy all through the fall. That winter, we wanted to go to the Boston Flower Show as we had done in our pre-cancer life. We liked to walk through the fantasy world of spring flowers, trees, running brooks, butterflies, and all the other insignia of spring artfully installed in the Expo Center. Going to the Flower Show was all the more wonderful because often we would need to battle a raging northeaster snowstorm to get there.

Every year we would take a tour of the major installations, and then look at the juried flower arrangements. Trudee always had her little notebook with her for recording the names of the more exotic plants on display. The idea was to plant them in our own yard. Most of the time, however, they were either impossible to find or too expensive to buy. The plants we could find, as it turned out, never did well. Still, hopes did spring eternal in that magical place so we never gave up the practice of carefully writing down the names of the plants that struck our fancy.

Then we would walk methodically up and down the dozen or so aisles on the more commercial side of the flower show. We collected brochures from contractors. We handled a water-filled plastic device guaranteed to make tomatoes grow earlier and larger. We ogled chrome and brass garden tools too good to use but beautiful to look at. Trudee would buy the latest in gardening gloves and yet more dahlia bulbs in hopes that I would be able to make these latest candidates grow. Stand after stand gave samples of honeys, spicy cheese mixes, very natural grain crackers, teas, jams, handmade soaps, dried flower arrangements, African violets. Already heavily laden, we would stop at the houseplant stall near the exit. We always bought something big, which we lugged back through the snow to the car and home.

The Flower Show of 1996 was different for us. The massive amounts of chemotherapy and progress of the disease itself were weakening Trudee. "I don't think I want to take the Evil Twin to the Flower Show," she said. "It's too hard for me to walk for all that time, and I don't think I can fight the crowds." As she spoke, I could see her also turning over the thought, "If I don't go now, when?"

It was a delicate negotiation between us and within each of us. We both recognized her physical limitations. We also recognized how much she wanted to go. "Let's go," I said. "We can walk a little and then find a place to sit for a while. We can get lunch there and rest. If it gets to be too much, we can go home." Trudee thought about that without saying much. A few days later, she floated the idea of renting a wheelchair. When I agreed that this sounded like an excellent idea, she pulled back a little. "We still have a few weeks. Let's think about it a little more."

There was a lot to think about. For Trudee, getting wheeled through the crowds signified major disability. Hair and appetite lost to chemotherapy can come back. Getting into the wheelchair felt like a lasting defeat. It meant that cancer was winning.

When we unloaded the wheelchair from the back of the car in the Expo Center parking lot, the snow was too deep for the chair to get through easily, so Trudee walked to the entrance while I pushed the chair. She sat down when we got inside, and we began to explore the exhibits. "We should have done this before," Trudee said. "Look how people are getting out of our way, and it's not just because you're driving like a madman." The wheelchair did open a path for us wherever we wanted to go. True, people refused to make eye contact with Trudee, but they did get out of our way. Then, just for a change, Trudee and I reversed places. I sat in the chair and she pushed me for a while. In short, we had fun. That fun was our way of resolving the dilemmas of our amphibian lives.

That same fall, we decided to buy a sailboat. That was another strategy for giving us a more singular life. Trudee and I had been going to the cottage on Cape Cod, at Sandy Neck, for fifteen years when she was diagnosed in July of 1994. Once we absorbed the shock of discovering that she had cancer, we decided to give up the cottage and to buy a sailboat. This was a big step for us. The cottage had been our home for so many summers that it was almost unthinkable not to go back to Sandy Neck for whatever summers might remain to us. Our friends in that little cluster of Cape Cod duck-hunting shacks were practically our family. We had lived through the cancer deaths of three of them already. Still, once we realized that our time together was sharply limited, Trudee and I wanted adventure more than we wanted security and familiarity.

Trudee wasn't feeling well at all the day we started looking in boatyards around Boston. It was hard for her to climb the ladder up into the boats standing in the yards. Most of the time, she sat down while I explored the boats and came back to describe what I had seen. I felt that our looking was more important than our reason for doing it. We were pretending that we had a future that could accommodate an adventure like a boat. I didn't think we would really find a boat that would suit us. I was sure that we were going through the motions in an elaborate game of self-deception. We would look and look, I thought, and then lose the sense of mission. "This must be a little crazy," I said. "Just keep looking," Trudee said. To my amazement, a friend found the perfect sailboat, and we bought it.

When I saw the boat, I knew it was the one for us. It was a real sailboat that could easily sleep four people, take Trudee and me to distant harbors, and be a summer home for us and our friends. The next weekend, Trudee and I drove down to Rhode Island where the boat was located to look at it together. "Buy it," she said without a moment's hesitation.

That was a decision that changed our lives. Having a new boat gave us all the details of boat ownership to think about. More important than the distraction, deciding to buy the boat defined for us in a very objective way just how we would lead our lives for the duration of our time together. It was one thing to hold in the abstract that we should not let the cancer get us down. It was quite another thing to actually make such a big commitment. The boat was a perfect focus. It pulled us into the future and it occupied our present with our sweet conversations about even the most mundane details of buying and owning a boat. Every aspect of this adventure was new to us.

Trudee and I then traveled around the coastal towns, looking for possible harbors to sail out of. Those trips were more physically difficult for Trudee than the earlier trips to explore boatyards had been. She had had more chemotherapy and was at times very weak. If we happened to hit low tide, the walkways down to the slips were so steep that she had a hard time walking back up. Still with infinite good will, patience, and inner strength, Trudee insisted on making these trips.

Even with the obvious limitations, these were wonderful outings for both of us. We visited little towns all up and down the coast. We enjoyed the time out of the house. More important, Trudee and I were acting as if we had a future. Maybe for the first time in our lives, we were living deliberately to create and design a future. We had to take the realities of our cancer life into consideration, but we were also working hard to make the most of what we had.

Finally, sailing together wasn't possible either. It was just too hard for Trudee to clamber into the boat and to keep her balance—even sitting—once we got under way. So we rented a house in Wellfleet on Cape Cod with friends for a week. The difference this time was that Trudee had no energy for walking the beach or climbing the dunes. We had to find things we could do while sitting down.

We armed ourselves with fresh white paper, drawing pencils, brushes, and two sets of watercolors. Neither of us had ever done anything like this. That wasn't the point. The point was that we had found an activity that we could do together, that would keep us connected with our world, that looked like fun. We never got very good at drawing or at watercolors. We never expected to learn technique. We just smeared our paints and got great satisfaction from looking closely at things and then sharing our crude representations of what we thought we saw. And we learned something, too, about how looking at the most commonplace things carefully changes us.

Hope and Fate

I can see how our ancestors got their idea of Fate. To the ancient Greeks, the Fates (Morai) were three old women spinning and cutting the thread of each person's life. Klotho (whose name comes from the Greek word for spinning) was the youngest of the women. She decided the moment of a person's birth. Lachesis (whose name comes from the Greek word to measure out) was also a spinner, but she presided over the future. The third Fate, Atropos (whose name comes from the Greek word for mute and inflexible), cut the thread into its allotted lengths. This she did without regard to age, sex, or social status. What she cut became a person's destiny. Today, thousands of years after those early philosophical concepts were invented, they still feel familiar. Living in the cancer world forces us back to those primitive questions because we are still dealing with those same questions and have no better answers.

Virtually everything in the cancer world pushes us toward a belief in destiny. We push from the border, across the arid plains, through the high mountain passes, into the peaceful valley until we reach our appointed destination. We may feel more passive than this. We may feel that we have our destiny to endure; and that we wait dumbly for our destiny to come. Survival in the cancer world depends upon cultivating a different sense of what is to come. *Destiny* is very different from *future*. The three old crones spin, assign, and cut. Future is a more congenial concept, coming from the Latin word for what is about to be (*futurus*). When we think of the future, we think of many possibilities from which one outcome will eventually happen. Destiny, on the other hand, is fixed. In the words of the novelist Graham Greene, "Hope is an instinct only the reasoning human mind can kill. An animal never knows despair."

Trudee and I could have crawled into any of the many dank caves we discovered in the cancer world. We could have taken refuge in depression and self-pity. Who would have criticized us for moping, considering the terrifying adventures we faced? We could have surrendered utterly to cancer and waited passively for our stretch of time to pass us by. We could have become angry and bitter. Instead, we recognized what the cancer could do to us and gave our energies to living as fully as we could for as long as we could. We hoped that if we lived for the moment, as much as we could without being outrageously irresponsible, the moments would accumulate to a pretty good pile.

Guessing What Our Partner Wants

The shrewd guess, the fertile hypothesis, the courageous leap to a tentative conclusion—these are the
most valuable coin of the thinker at work.

—*Jerome S. Bruner,*
The Process of Education

People living in the cancer world believe that cancer has thrust
them into an experience so totally new and bizarre that it
demands radically new ways of thinking, feeling, and acting. Anxiety
changes the coloring of the most familiar situations so that we barely
recognize them. Details jump into prominence that ordinarily would
be background noise. Before we entered the cancer world, for example, if our partner came home from the dentist with a swollen and
painful mouth, we would be sympathetic, but we wouldn't be overwhelmed by the terror. We knew that the pain would pass, and that
some long-term good would come from the temporary discomfort.
In the cancer world, however, we rush to do something about pain or
loss of appetite or difficulty sleeping or weakness or fear or depression.

Eating is a good example of how something that normally stays in
the background gets a lot of attention in the cancer world. If our
partner skipped a meal in the pre-cancer life, it would mean that he
just wasn't hungry, or something else just as benign. In the cancer
world, not eating could be because of anything from post-treatment
queasiness to horrible pain, and much in between. In the pre-cancer
world, time usually took care of the matter. In the cancer world, there
is no time. When Trudee's appetite waned, I saw it as a sign that she

was losing her will to live. I would immediately imagine malnutrition and all its complications. Sometimes loss of appetite is a serious problem to be dealt with medically, and fortunately, medications are available for controlling nausea and pain and for stimulating appetite. But not every uneaten meal is a signal of disaster.

As with so many other things in the cancer life, we see what looks like a problem and then try to guess how we can help our partner solve it. If our view of the cancer life is clear, we can guess solutions to the problems of living with cancer. If our view is confused about what we want to be doing or think we should be doing, we may never discover those solutions. Getting our partner to eat, for example, can quickly become an issue far bigger than the eating itself. People who are going through chemotherapy or radiation therapy are sick, worried, and no longer physically active; in fact, many of the people in the cancer world have little or no interest in food. The sight of food—the smell, the thought of sitting at the table—is enough to disgust them. The important thing to remember is that *they* know how they feel. Who are we to say, "Just try this. I know you'll like it"? We must be careful not to make the issue of food into a struggle over who controls their body.

Cancer is very different when seen from the two points of view within the cancer partnership. As with the example of food, this difference in views can create problems. There are moments in the cancer life when we are forced to realize that we and our partner are quite different people, separated by our common experiences in the cancer world.

We are thus fooling ourselves if we think we know the other person's innermost life. Although we both live in the cancer world and participate in many aspects of that cancer life together, we are not the partner who has the cancer. Trudee, for example, may have been feeling profoundly fatigued and weak after a cycle of chemotherapy, while people around her were telling her how good she looked. When she didn't set the record straight, the rest of us were more than willing to believe that her pain was not so bad anymore and that she was getting her energy back. In fact, Trudee may have felt that other people just didn't want to hear her complain, or she may have been depressed, or she may have been too tired to correct people's misconception, or she may have been motivated by a host of inexplicable feelings that were hers alone.

I could never really know the innermost life of Trudee, of course, but still I had to act. I often had to do something despite my very imperfect knowledge of what she was feeling, what she really wanted, what would have been good for her whether she knew it or not. This is the part of the cancer life that is surprisingly like falling in love. Like romantic love, it is a life that succeeds only by our making good guesses about what the other person wants. The other person is pretty much a mystery, even in the best of times. But in good times, we can make some easy guesses and get credit for trying. Maybe they should have been anemones instead of roses, but the idea of giving her flowers was a good one. Still, as in the cancer world, the stakes in the world of romantic love can be high. Enough missed guesses and he may be gone; she may lose interest. The poet Friedrich Schiller wrote, "If you want to understand others, look into your own heart." This works, up to a point. The trick in making the proper love guesses is to start in your own heart, but not to make that other person yourself. This is especially true in the cancer world, because it is such a strange world and because the stakes are almost prohibitively high.

Thus, playing the role of cancer partner means understanding what the other person wants. This demands an inspired guess on our part and a courageous leap to put that hypothesis to the test. This is not very different from the lover's guess of what will be funny, emotionally right, sensual, interesting, or satisfying to the other person. The guess may turn out to be wrong, but without the attempt, there is nothing.

Guessing how to be with the other person and what to do for the person is made even more difficult by the fact that living in the cancer world changes people. Couples in the cancer world are rarely at the same place and at the same stage in their acceptance of the disease and their adaptation to the changes cancer has made in their lives. It is almost predictable that when treatment ends, the person with cancer immediately starts to feel worse emotionally, while the partner starts to feel better. The two people are in very different places. During treatment, they are so focused on the treatment that the fears and anxieties about the disease are put aside. When the treatment ends, they have to start dealing with what the disease means. The people with cancer feel more vulnerable and more anxious about survival than ever before. Partners, in contrast, think that their lives can finally get back to normal.

Survival in that atmosphere is the goal of the partners with cancer. We, the other partners, may not think that survival itself is our prime concern. We are often more interested in protecting the status quo.

Although without a doubt, our partner's death is the greatest threat to our own status quo, we seem to pay less attention to this stark reality than to some of the more manageable aspects of life in the cancer world. We partners are thus often the champions of a return to normalcy. Even in the stifling atmosphere of the cave, more than anything, we dream of regaining our former lives. We want to go back across that boundary and re-enter the world of innocence that we used to inhabit. We are sure that once our partner's treatment is finished, our lives will quickly fall back into the pre-cancer life we remember so fondly. Our partners will resume their former roles immediately, and we will be able to relax from the rigors of the cancer life.

Talking to each other helps nail down some of the ambiguities of what the other person wants, but not all of them. Someone can say "Please give me a drink of water" or "I am worried about the results of those tests" or "I want to go to Minneapolis because . . . ." But we are lucky when our cancer partners can tell us so explicitly what they want. Most of the time, their needs are so personal, their reasons so entangled, and their feelings so subterranean, it is impossible for us to guess what they mean. We may therefore pass each other in the cancer world without making serious contact.

The Silence

One of the risks of the cancer life is that of falling into the silence that can eat at the heart of the partnership. This silence is corrosive, and very different from the shared quiet that can hold partners together. "The moment that I felt closest to my wife was the moment of her diagnosis," a partner told me. "We both felt the blow together. From that point on, however, I could feel the defense mechanisms kick in to separate us from each other. In our loneliness, we felt the blow separately." A similar separation happened to another cancer partner. "I remember the wonderful night talks my husband and I used to have at the beginning," she told me. "We could share our fears and listen to each other's hopes. I missed them terribly when my husband began to withdraw from me into his own cancer world. We had always shared everything before that."

A man I met said that his wife withdrew into herself and became depressed after a recurrence of her stomach cancer. "She got so distant from me that I couldn't reach her any more," he said. "She still wanted me to do things for her, but she never gave me a clue as to what she might want. The more she got depressed, the more she pulled away from me, and the more I got depressed and angry. I couldn't believe that I ever loved this woman. And the more angry and frustrated I got, the less I could guess what she wanted of me. Eventually, I even stopped trying."

One cancer partner told me that the weight of his wife's disease was overwhelming. "I don't want her to be alone, feeling that she is the only one in this place of depression. So sometimes I deliberately put myself in the same place of depression. Not together with her, but separately in the same place. As a result, I feel like I am left alone in my own depression and she is just as isolated in hers. She wants me to help, she wants me to be there for her and I want to be there with her. But I can't because it is very difficult to get through that force field of hers to the real eye of the storm."

Another cancer partner told me he feels enormous pressure when he and his wife are not talking. "She doesn't tell me where she is. Although I try to feel what she must be feeling, I know that I don't live with her multiple myeloma every second the way she does. She could make it a little easier for me by giving me a hint of what she might want from me. I know that she is alone in this horrible place with no way to vent her desperation and frustration. I don't want her to be alone in that place where she can't do anything to release herself. I want to get into her mind so that I can do whatever will help her find some relief. That is the center of the experience for me—trying to figure out how my wife and I can work together so that I am not forced into playing both parts. I have to be hopeful and confident, but at some point I just have to give that up and say to myself, 'This is really horrible and desperate and I can't believe what's going on here.' I can only say that to myself because she would fall apart if she suspected that I was thinking this way. Instead, we don't say anything."

Guessing

Our guesses are probes into the silence. Many things are going on in the minds of our cancer partners that are only dimly apparent to us. For example, many partners with cancer go through the routine that

Trudee enacted with me over and over: She would pick out my next wife. We would be stopped at a red light with a stream of pedestrians passing in front of the car. If a woman walked in front of us, less than half my age, with a skin-tight skirt only slightly wider than her belt, orange spiked hair, maybe a tattoo on her arm, and a row of rings stuck in her lower lip, Trudee would say, "There's your next wife." I never really knew what she was thinking, but she did this routine so often, I finally had to ask her to stop. I told her I didn't think the joke was funny.

A cancer partner told me that her husband picked out her next mate, too. "He will be blond, very, very pale, short, and a heavy smoker. Everything I don't like in a man," he told her. Her husband also told a friend of his to make sure that his wife married the kind of man that he had picked out. "But my husband has also stipulated that his friend has to live longer than I do in order to make sure that I am buried with him, my present husband, and not with the short, blond smoker."

Perhaps there is an explanation for this apparently common occurence in the cancer world: In Gail Godwin's novel *The Good Husband*, Magda Danvers, who has recently come home after surgery for her cancer ("the Great Uncouth," as she calls it), imagines her husband Francis's next wife. When he objects to her cavalier attitude, she answers seriously, "We might as well have some fun over your future while I'm still here to enjoy it with you." "But I don't enjoy imagining life without you," he tells her. "But, I told you," she responds. "My imagining it with you now is a way of keeping company with you after I'm gone."

This logic is not immediately obvious.

It takes a great leap of insight to jump into the other person's cancer world. One night, a cancer partner and his family were watching a television news show. His wife's advanced breast cancer had severely weakened her and was causing her a great deal of pain. She lay on the couch while the others sat around her. The television report was about an older man with cancer who was being cared for at home by his adult children and a hospice nurse. The point of the report was that the hospice nurse was stealing the old man's morphine for her own use. His children suspected that the nurse was stealing the morphine so they filled the morphine bottle with Ipecac. When the nurse went into the bathroom with what she thought was the bottle of morphine, the children locked the door and called the police. "The four of us were howling in laughter at the chutzpah of those people. Suddenly I noticed that my wife was crying. She was looking behind the interviewer and the man's son to where the poor sick man was sitting on his bed in a stark, barren room. There was nothing in his little room, no flowers, nothing that would give any life to the room at all. My wife was seeing right through the scene to the sick man on his bed. She said, 'This is not what I want for myself.'" His wife was crying and shaking with fear. While he held her, he was mad at himself for not protecting her from the agony of the story they had just watched. "I thought I was being very uncaring to be laughing at something that made her so sad."

Months passed. The cancer partner's wife developed unremitting fears of being overpowered and defenseless. She felt raw terror almost all the time. One time, she was very agitated and kept saying, 'Don't put me downstairs. I don't want to be locked in a little room with no flowers.' Her eyes were big, and she was breathing hard, short breaths. "After an agonizing time, I realized that she was talking about the television report we had watched together months earlier. I opened the door to our backyard and had her look at the bright sun and how it was shining into her room. 'There's your flower bed that we planted last summer,' I said to her. 'Look at the vase full of flowers on your bureau. You've got the sunshine and the flowers. Until the day you die,' I said, 'you will always be surrounded by both.' She became calm again.

Distortions are an inevitable consequence of living in the cancer world because the cancer world is in part a mental world of our own making. It is full of mirages and other illusions. Our partners don't always know what they want from us. It would be asking a lot to expect them to think clearly enough to explain to us what they would like us to do. These are difficult and frightening times. Pain and fear— not to mention the effects of treatment and the various drugs used to minimize the unpleasant effects of treatment—cloud their thinking and confuse their feelings.

We need to be willing to take some big risks ourselves. We need to volunteer things, we need to hazard guesses. Although rejection was often frustrating if what I offered to Trudee wasn't right for the moment, I didn't take the rejection personally. I thought it would be unfair to Trudee, sick and weak and scared, to also impose on her the burden of telling me what I should be doing for her.

Doing What We Can

Before the cancer, when Trudee would ask me to do something around the house or to pick up something at the grocery store, I was happy enough to do her such a small favor. Often she could have done the errand for herself, but it was easier for her to have me do it. If an expression of slight impatience flitted across my face, which I must admit did happen from time to time, she adopted her most reproving tone and delivered the mini-lecture: "Well, this is a doo-fer relationship, you know. You do for me, and I do for you. Other-wise, I'm out of here." Cancer changed all that. When Trudee asked me to do things, they were things she could no longer do for herself without a great and painful effort. If she *could* do something, she insisted on doing it for herself.

Of course I took care of Trudee. When she had no appetite, I searched the supermarket and specialty food shops for foods that would hopefully appeal to her. When she needed help climbing the stairs, I gave her some added muscle and balance from behind. When she needed me to keep the Trudee News Network (TNN) going, I made telephone calls to relatives and friends.

Some of the mundane tasks that are so necessary in the cancer world became joint exercises in caring. Her injections, for instance. For about ten days after each round of chemotherapy, she would need to give herself a daily injection of GCSF, a drug that stimulates the growth of white blood cells. For some reason, Trudee was very inse-cure about filling the syringe. I think she was nervous about drawing precisely the right amount of medicine. Whatever her reason for not wanting to set up her injection, I welcomed the chance to participate in her treatment. Nights when she needed her shot, just before bed-time I would go through the same routine: After washing my hands, I would get a large dinner plate from the kitchen cabinet and the GCSF from the refrigerator. I would carry these things upstairs to Trudee with a combination of feelings: satisfaction that we were doing some-thing positive and doing it well, reverence for her efforts, hope that the treatment would work, and relief that this somewhat complex and ini-tially forbidding procedure had become familiar. If this part of the can-cer could become familiar, I thought, maybe the whole thing would.

Once upstairs, I would wipe the dinner plate with an alcohol wipe (always in circles from the center to the periphery, as we had been taught by the nurse at the Dana-Farber Cancer Institute) to provide a clean work surface for putting the syringe together. Once I had the needle and syringe assembled and filled the syringe with GCSF, I handed the syringe to Trudee along with two alcohol wipes. She gave herself the shot. Every shot night, she would say "thank you" to me and I would reply, "No, no. Thank *you.*"

The partners with cancer may assume all too readily that they are a burden to others. It takes a strong sense of perspective to *not* think this way because it is an easy assumption to make. The partner with cancer must go through a whole gamut of unpleasant and unwanted experiences. There may be little choice because the unpleasant treatments promise some relief. The partner with cancer then may look at the other partner and reason that one of them is stuck with the cancer fate, but that the other partner is free to choose a more congenial one. The reasonable choice would be to escape the cancer world altogether. "Are we having fun yet?" Trudee would ask me as she lay on the hospital bed getting her chemotherapy.

Of course, everybody would like to escape back across the border to the pre-cancer world. Huddled together in the lee of a rock, trying to get some shelter from the bone-chilling blasts that make the highlands of the cancer world almost impassable, the partner with cancer says, "You wouldn't be here if it weren't for me." If the obvious choice is to flee and yet the partner stays in the cancer world, then, so reasons the partner with cancer, staying in that world of anguish and pain must be a burden. Indeed, Trudee never stopped apologizing for making me go through such unpleasantness.

What *Does* the Other Want?

The more we try to make those inspired guesses about what our partner might want, the better we get at it. As we get better, we get closer because each guess, each leap to a tentative conclusion about what might be a good thing to do, adds a strand in the knot of love. It is very gratifying when we make the right guess. But it is important that we also prepare ourselves to be wrong. If we actually ask our partners what they want from us, we may be surprised to find that we are only approximately right. I met many people in my travels in the cancer world, and I asked them what they wanted from their partners. This is what some of them told me.

Sy
Diagnosis: Advanced prostate cancer
Age: 56

What do we want? We want to spend as much time as we can having fun. Sometimes our humor is a little black, but it's still laughing. The big joke in our cancer support group is that someone's spouse wants to put more money into the IRA for retirement. I say, What for? Take the money and do something.

My wife and I have been traveling a lot. We went into a luggage store with two other couples to buy a suitcase for a trip we were about to take. The salesman began to sing the praises of a piece of luggage he was showing us. "This bag is bulletproof," he said. "No bullet can get through it, and if it does, the fabric just heals itself up again. And that's not all," he said, "this bag has a lifetime guarantee." At that, my friend asked him with a straight face as he looked at me, "Whose life?" Four of us fell apart in giggles, while the other couple with us was awkwardly silent. They were absolutely scandalized that we could make such a crude joke about my prostate cancer.

What do we want? We want other people to share some of the burden of our diagnosis. If they can laugh with us, they are sharing that burden.

I also want my wife to be close to me. One time, I was in a really bad way. I had a three-week stay in the hospital, near the beginning of my treatment. I knew I was sick, but I didn't know at the time how very sick I was. My wife was staying with friends near the hospital. Every morning she would come to the hospital, always at the same time. I would get up at three or four in the morning and watch the clock until she arrived. By seven-thirty, I was really looking for her. One day, she didn't show up. I was furious and frightened. When she finally walked in two hours late, I was all over her case. As it turned out, there had been a big accident on the bridge between where she was staying and the hospital. An oil truck had turned over and exploded. The whole bridge was in flames. There was no way she could get to the hospital until they put out the fire and cleared the wreckage. When I found out what had happened, I felt bad for yelling at her. But I really needed her to be with me that morning. What did I need from her? It wasn't anything specific. I just wanted her to be there with me.

When my condition was desperate, she didn't need to ask me what I needed, and I didn't need to say anything. She just knew. During the intermediate times, when I wasn't so desperate, I had to think of whether I could get through those times without her. If I was just feeling lonely, I wouldn't ask her to keep me company. If she asked me how I was doing, I would just tell her that I was fine. I would run a judgment on my pain or my fear. Then I would ask myself, according to my own internal standard, "Is it worth having me ask her specifically for this kind of help or is this something that I can just hope she notices?" Sometimes, I might have a need, but think it was just too silly to ask for. So a lot of the time, I was needing her attention, for big things or small, just hoping that she would notice. Sometimes she did and sometimes she didn't.

My wife has also been very important in grounding me. I still bounce my fears off her, the crazy thoughts that are running through my mind. I need to check whether these are just my mind running away with terrors, or whether this is a real thing to worry about. I trust her judgment completely because I question my own. But I can't talk to her about everything that goes through my mind. I am sometimes afraid that she'll think I'm silly. But a lot of times, it's the silly things that bother me the most. I remember one time I needed a colonoscopy, and just reading the informed consent was enough to throw me into a panic. I couldn't sign the form. I had to have the nurse bring my wife in from the waiting room to help me. She came in and said to me, as only she could, "You big ass. Roll over and let them do the damn thing. This is ridiculous." I know that sounds harsh, but she really helped me get through a very hard time. She brought me back to reality.

Terri
Diagnosis: Metastatic breast cancer
Age: 47

When I was first diagnosed with breast cancer, my husband and I were very close. It was one of the few times in our lives when I saw him just burst into tears. It was so sad. I was too sick to be able to give him any comfort. I was too overwhelmed to take care of him. Then we grew apart a little. There is now a certain amount of detachment because of my own uncertainty about what's going on with me. If the situation is emotionally charged, I will strike out. I don't want to do that. So I would rather he gave me a little more emotional space.

I don't know what I need. In our life, it was always my kids first, always my husband first. You get cancer, and all of a sudden you're first. My husband doesn't like that adjustment. He likes to have me mother him. If I'm not feeling well, he can feel when I'm withdrawing. That's the worst part of having cancer. You lose the ability to love and to care for other people. When I see my husband's pain like that, I want to take it away. But there is no way I can take it away because I am responsible for causing this horrendous, painful situation. It is the cancer that is causing the loss of the life that we had together, but it is *my* cancer.

It's a terrible predicament to try to come together as a couple when our life is fractured so badly and the outcome isn't known. There was a chance that my breast cancer was gone completely. Then it came back, with a whole new set of much scarier rules. I see the reality that this can kill you. Before you could say to yourself, "This is an illness that can be terminal but you'll be lucky. You'll beat it." That's how we got through it the first time. We said, "All right, we're going to do everything we're supposed to do. Then we'll see if we will be lucky or not lucky." When the cancer came back, it felt as if the answer to our question was, "Not lucky."

As my treatment goes on and I can relax a little bit into being a person with cancer, I am becoming more aware of what I need from my husband. The biggest thing that I need from him right now is to be allowed to say what is on my mind, whether it is something that is very scary about the cancer or something that strikes me as funny. People with cancer deal with a lot of scary stuff, so most of what I want my husband to listen to is scary stuff. It's too much of a burden for me to be in one of those don't-talk, don't-ask things with him. Then I have second thoughts. I think that this may not be entirely fair to him. I need to figure out whether it is really necessary to burden him with the pain that I'm going through. I can only assume that he is going through his own pain, and that his and mine are probably pretty similar. If we could share that pain, maybe we both would be a little better. But I don't know. Maybe his pain is completely different from mine.

Listening to the hard stuff scares the hell out of my husband. I was always the happy-go-lucky one in our relationship. I always made a joke out of things. Now if I start getting serious about my cancer—especially if I start crying—it scares the shit out of him. After three years of living with my cancer, he is just now starting to learn that I will be OK after I get the scary stuff out into the open. That is the most important part because until you share the really scary, ugly fears (even physically how dying is going to happen) and talk about pain, you're locked alone into the horror. I need to be able to say, "This is what is going on in my mind, and how do you feel about it?" I don't think he is comfortable with that.

If the two of us talked about this real threat, where nothing is imagined, it wouldn't become a mental health issue but rather a very objective problem that has a lot of emotional baggage with it. It would be a real problem. But if I do that, and then I hear an answer from him that doesn't sound friendly, I just pick up my ball and I go home. My husband's answer to my anxieties about upcoming CT scans and the next treatment, for example, is "Well, just don't think about it. Don't let it overwhelm you." That answer shuts me down. I would prefer that he confirm that it's scary for me. That's all. I would be liberated from the feeling that I was just being neurotic.

My husband could also be more active. Whenever there's a crisis, he does fine. Everything gets done well. Things that need doing get done, emotions get handled. He's just there. But maybe he and I have different scales for what a crisis is. If I think it's a crisis and he doesn't, then I'm not going to get what I need. Why should he mobilize if he thinks it isn't a crisis? On the other hand, why isn't he mobilized if *I* think it is a crisis? Maybe I should say to him, "You may not think this is a crisis, but I do."

There are times when we can slip into the dark side when we don't need to and we could be pulled out. Not that he has the responsibility for rescuing me from my own fears (nobody has that responsibility), but he could help me.

I like to joke about it, and he doesn't. He seems to feel that if he joked about my fears or about the cancer, he might make the worst fears happen. He's not comfortable with joking. So I have to make the cancer experience comfortable for him so that he doesn't drive me away. It stops me from finding out what *my* fears are if my husband doesn't want to start on that journey with me.

I want to feel that I am allowed to say anything I want. The allowing part comes from allowing myself to express myself without having to worry about the people-pleasing aspect of my life. Throughout my whole life, I was always concerned about how other people thought about me. That's the first thing to go when you get cancer. You don't have to worry about making other people feel good. In some ways, it is really exciting to be able to focus on the ugly part of it. Then reality isn't quite as bad as what we imagined, hopefully.

Felicia
Diagnosis: Lymphoma
Age: 63

Cancer is part of your identity. I am a mother and a wife and a working woman, and cancer is also part of who I am. When people interact with me, I expect them to recognize the fact that I have been through fourteen years of a very difficult time. I appreciate it when a person asks me what I have done all these years to keep myself going. I feel that they are genuinely interested in me, not just in my disease.

I want to surround myself with people who can let me express my feelings instead of putting them down. I don't fear death, but like all cancer patients, I fear the last months of life, when things can get really painful or bad physically. I think that is what we are all worried about. If I say something about my fear of death or worries about getting sick again, I don't want somebody to tell me that those feelings are ridiculous. I don't want anyone to tell me that this next operation will be my last operation because I know that that is not true. I have already been through fourteen years of operations.

I want somebody to just be able to listen to me and maybe not even say anything, but just to give me a time and place to let it out. A little hug and a little physical attention at times and to be treated a little bit special for what I have been going through. I would like to be pampered a little bit. I think everybody wants that.

I have sought out other cancer patients over the years, and they are wonderful support. They truly are the ones I can turn to if I am anxious about a CT scan coming up. I call one of my cancer friends rather than one of my "normal" friends. Within five minutes of talking with one of these cancer friends, I know that I am being understood. I may not be perfectly calm after talking with them, but it certainly helps a lot.

There are things that I won't discuss with my normal friends. They just don't understand the language. I also don't want to impose on them too much. Friends who are going through life in the normal way might say that I am getting awfully depressing. So I don't talk to these normal friends much about the cancer. My difficulty with these normal friends is that they tend to talk about trivial things. I am amazed that these things can trouble them. I feel that I am on the outside looking in on a world where I don't belong anymore. I don't talk about retirement. I don't care about redecorating my house. It is painful being in their company because they are truly planning for old age. I am not there. For me next month is almost coming into reality. Beyond that is too far into the future for me to deal with.

For me, support is somebody being able to listen, somebody giving me physical attention and treating me like a princess, and validating what I am saying by not putting down my thoughts and feelings. Support is saying, "I can't really feel what you are feeling, but I can hear what you are saying" instead of saying "You're ridiculous. You're crazy."

There was a stage show recently by a young man who had lymphoma at the age of twenty-two. I cried and laughed hysterically at some of the things in the show. When I went home, I told my husband about the show and about how funny parts of it were. He said, "How could you laugh at that? I couldn't have gone with you because it would have been so depressing." Yet laughing about things is a sign of how we have accepted the cancer. People who haven't had it can't get the joke. For me, living with my husband is like living with a person who just doesn't get the joke. When you try to explain to someone why a joke is funny, you realize just how different the two of you are. Since my husband is a physician, we can talk the medical talk. We can analyze the scientific literature, we can talk about the doctors. He wouldn't get into the other sides of my cancer though.

One of our big dilemmas is that from the time of my diagnosis fourteen years ago, I have been in some kind of support system. At first there were no cancer support groups except for breast cancer. I was told that my only choice was to go to a psychiatrist. I did, but the psychiatrist didn't have cancer. Over the years, I evolved to an understanding of my cancer. Support groups have developed. But my husband has done nothing all those years. It is very difficult when one person stands still and is the same as back then and the other person has evolved and has come into a different place. That other person is left behind. He and I really speak different languages.

It drives him crazy that cancer is such an important part of my identity. I have cancer friends on the computer. I turn the computer on once a day to get my e-mail from them, to check on what's going on. He screamed at me the other day, "Can't you go one day without checking to see what they're saying about cancer? Can't you just put it behind you for a little while? What is this obsession?" I said to him, "I'm not obsessed. I function. These cancer friends are good friends of mine and I want to hear what they are saying." I feel an obligation to help others if I can. We help each other.

I suggested that my husband join a support group for the spouses of people with cancer. First he made excuses: I have to work that night; I have tickets to a ball game. I realized that he didn't want to go. He said it would be too depressing to be in a room with other people whose spouses are sick and dying. I told him that it is not depressing for me, and I'm the one who is approaching death. Why would it be depressing for him? I said, "Do it for me." He refused. He says that he would be afraid to say in public that he hates my cancer and that he sometimes wishes that the whole thing could be over. He says he would be embarrassed to say anything like that.

Because my husband is dealing with it so poorly and hasn't worked on living with my cancer, there is so much frustration and anger that he will lash out at me. It is very hurtful. He said to me, "Look what you've done to fourteen years of my life. You are so selfish. All you can think about is yourself. Do you realize that there are two people involved in your cancer? You never think about me."

But I am not a clinging wife who asks him to rub my back. I turn to other people because I can't turn to him. Him calling me selfish has gotten me the angriest. I understand that he has needs. He has to work on them himself. He also falls apart every time I have a recurrence. He is very pessimistic. I told him that I would keep myself going if I have another recurrence. I'll turn to my support system because I don't expect him to support me. He hasn't been able to. But I can't be his support at those times. I need all the energy I can get for myself.

We have discussed divorce. He said to me, "Don't you dare do that. If we got divorced at this point, everybody would look at me and say that I wasn't able to deal with your cancer." He was so concerned that he would be embarrassed. In fact, he has given up. When I'm sick and I come home from the hospital, my husband either isn't there for me at all or he calls my sister to come from Florida and take care of me. After my operation a month ago, he left town for a week. His comment before he went away was, "You do very fine without me. You're so independent, you don't need me anyway." I feel badly for him. I said to him, "After I'm gone, you'll be living many more years. You really need to address these issues. They are not going to go away." The more he is that way, the more distant I become. When I came home from the hospital, he still had two more days before he came home. My friends took care of me. When he came home he said, "Now you're going to throw this up to me because I wasn't home when you got out of the hospital." I can't deal with it. He just has so many problems.

Talking with the doctors about some pretty serious stuff, I started to cry. My husband just sat there, two chairs away from me. He became more uncomfortable. I felt so sad for him that he couldn't show his concern for me. He couldn't just get up and come over to me to give some comfort. So I would prefer that he not come. He never looked at my CT scans or x-rays, even though the doctors invited him to do so. I have too many things to do for myself to spend time being my husband's psychiatrist. I've got the cancer problem and I've got the husband problem. For me to improve things for him, now, I would have to give up the identity that I have developed for myself over all these years. I'm not going to give up my independence and the way I'm dealing with my cancer.

Ben
Diagnosis: Orbital carcinoma
Age: 39

I don't want pity. I want to be loved. Pity is "Oh, poor you. This must be awful. I feel badly for you. How can you go on?" Thanks. That's just what I do *not* need. People have said that I am being so brave. I take pride in it. I feel that I have dealt with this well. If people are acknowledging that, I will take their statement at face value and believe that they are being sincere and that it is not just a code for pity.

I keep dichotomizing the world into those people like me with cancer and those people without it. It is probably not quite so black and white, but people with cancer often say that it is easier for them than for the people who support them. There are things that the cancer patient doesn't have to deal with, and there are more resources and more societal norms to fit into roles for the person with cancer. If we are looking for how to behave, we have models already formed for us. For the people who support us, there is more ambiguity.

The other thing that makes it easier is that the cancer patient often is allowed to just concentrate on getting as well as possible. Everyone understands that that is an OK preoccupation to retreat into. Not only is there not an equivalent thing for the partner to concentrate on, but the partner also is left to pick up the pieces of what the cancer patient is not doing because he is concentrating on his own situation. The partner has to do extra things on top of having to deal with the potential loss of the cancer patient and the constant worries.

I am now in a space where I hope the cancer doesn't come back. I have gone through my treatments, and now I look forward to the reconstructive surgery to put my face back together. Basically, I am back on my feet. So I am now trying to return to living a normal life. When I was in the middle of my treatments, I was focusing on getting better. Even through that period, I tried to keep things as normal as possible. I worked, even though I probably should not have. I tried to maintain the life I had before and the life I wanted to lead. Through this entire time, I tried to at least acknowledge and give legitimacy to my wife's feelings and to recognize her burdens. I recognized the legitimacy of her feeling burdened. Not that I *was* a burden. We both had to go through this: Letting myself and letting ourselves allow the community to see us in our vulnerable state. The synagogue, which is our primary social community, and the religious school worked out a program to help us, especially preparing meals, but not only that. As we were muddling through, it was good to let people who knew us and loved us into our lives to help.

I want my wife's logistical help. That is very important because there are things I cannot do for myself. I want her to continue to see me as her husband and not as her cancer-patient partner. I want to preserve the conditions of our prior relationship. I want her to treat me as she has always treated me. I recognize that things are different, but I don't want to be seen as a pitiable thing. I don't want pity to be the main way that she identifies with me.

The other thing I want from her, and this has been the source of our greatest tension, is to be as positive as she can be. I am a natural optimist. I recognize that my wife is a worrier. This was an issue exacerbated by the cancer, not created by it. She is the child of Holocaust survivors and grew up with the knowledge that things can get horrible quickly. That has always been an undercurrent in her life, and now that this has happened, she sees some justification for that worldview.

She was also a literature major in college, and sometimes she sees these things in terms of literary designs. One of the ways she tries to make sense of all this is to put together a design in which this all fits. It doesn't fit, of course. It comes back to what do we do with where we are now. We need to go forward rather than worrying about what has already been. It is really *how* we go forward. We have to support each other. We each have our own things that we are dealing with. To get through this together, we need to help each other.

I have changed my attitude. At the beginning, I wanted to focus on just dealing with the medical part of it by myself. I wanted to concentrate on inner strength and making medical decisions myself. My wife quite naturally wanted to be with me through all this. At the beginning, I was grudgingly tolerating that. I felt, of course, that she had a right to be there. My attitude was that if I have something to deal with, I want to deal with it by myself, even though the other person involved is my wife. That was especially true of the medical decisions. Partly, I didn't want her to worry. There was a little feeling of wanting to protect her. It was really that I wanted to deal with it myself. I couldn't just tell her not to come because we didn't have that kind of marriage.

Then two things became obvious to me. One was that, whether she was right by my side or at home while I was at the doctor, she was going to have anxieties. In fact, I realized that it would reduce her anxieties to be with me and to hear directly from the doctor what the information was. We still had different takes on what the doctor told us, but her anxieties were less for being there. So I was doing myself a favor from that perspective. The other thing was that she would hear things that I missed that were important in reaching a medical decision. For something so complex and with such ambiguity about the right way to do things, it is impossible to hear it through the filter of my own anxiety. So I moved on the medical stuff toward letting her help me. And the emotional sides of things are intertwined with everything else.

What really helped there was the group at the Wellness Community. Hearing how people on each of our sides of the fence dealt with the cancer and to talk about it together gave us more and more a sense of seeing things from the other perspective. That brought us closer together. It took the freakishness out of it. My tendency is to want to be given space to deal with things. So for a while, I didn't want to talk about it too much. I just wanted to focus on working things out in my mind. I wanted to talk about it when things were uncertain, but basically I wanted to rely on myself. My wife is different. She wants to work things out openly. She wants to bounce ideas off left and right and be totally communicative, especially when things are not certain. I realized that if we take the Golden Rule, do unto others as you would have others do unto you, we were both doing what the other did *not* want done. We both had to recognize that and to acknowledge the needs of the other.

I don't get annoyed now when she talks about it, and she picks her times more carefully for talking with me. Now I give her legitimate releases rather than resisting every time she brings it up. There is an ebb and flow now whereas before it was more like water and oil.

Hard Questions

I wish I could say that Trudee was any less a mystery to me than these people were to their partners. I wish I could say that I asked her directly what she wanted of me as I had asked these people what they wanted of their partners. I didn't ask her; and I doubt that many partners engaged in the struggle to keep going in the cancer world would ask. Now that I think about it, it seems so sensible to just ask. But, as in the happier moments of romance, this tactic is only moderately successful. Assuming the risk of making a guess seems to be valuable.

After her diagnosis, Trudee would often ask me hard questions, and sometimes she would ask me impossible questions. If she asked me whether I thought treatment A might be better than treatment

B, for example, I would try to find out. If she wanted to know what the medical literature said about survival rates for people with her kind of cancer, painful as it was to do, I would search the literature and we would discuss what I had learned. These questions were hard to think about, but they weren't the impossible questions.

The impossible questions took a lot of learning on my part before I knew what to do with them. If Trudee had said, "Don't you think we should rewrite our wills?" the right thing for me to do would be to call a lawyer. The wrong thing would have been to sit down next to her, reassuringly hold her hand and say, "Why? We've got plenty of good years ahead of us."

I learned to distinguish Trudee's impossible questions from her hard ones by watching her respond to my answers. No matter how I applied myself to answer her really difficult questions, I could see that sometimes my answers were not satisfying her. In time I realized that she wasn't asking those questions to get my answers. She knew I couldn't answer a question like "Do you think I'm going to die this year?" Nobody could know the answers to a question like that. She wasn't looking for an answer; she wanted to hear from somebody she trusted that her fears were valid. In our innocent pre-cancer life, I probably would have said something like "Oh, don't be silly. Of course you are going to be OK." The cancer life prohibits such evasions. Breaking the trust with half answers is the surest way to find yourselves making separate passages through the cancer world.

Trudee's impossible questions were requests for emotional support, not requests for answers of fact. There are plenty of "facts," of course, like the numbers that come back after a blood test. Those facts are objective statements of something that got counted or measured. Other "facts" are like the life expectancy tables for people with various kinds of cancer. Those facts are statements of probabilities that apply to groups of people but not to any individual in particular. Still other "facts" are the images captured by the CT scan and the MRI. They show what is actually there. If the cancer world were only a place of fact, playing the role of the cancer partner would be far easier than it is in actual practice. It is not just a place of simple fact.

These facts are all objective in their way. But even the images aren't as objective as one might think. For almost two years, Trudee's scans showed that she had tumors in less than half her liver. This was bad but not disastrous because the liver is a very redundant organ, and Trudee's liver was working fine. She had no symptoms, so we didn't think there was any reason to worry. Then some time in the second year, Trudee had an MRI. This much more sensitive imaging technique showed that at least 80 percent of her liver was affected. Suddenly, we had a new reality. She hadn't changed, but our view of things did.

Life in the cancer world is based on objective facts like these, but they are colored by what we make of them. The facts don't mean anything until we interpret them. As a result, the cancer world is very a much a life that we create. Despite the real caves, deserts, rivers, mountains, the gloom and the searing light of the cancer world, our real life in the cancer world is born of both what we see there and what we make of it. We cancer partners must be in close touch with each other throughout our travels in the cancer world lest we become separated in each our own mental cancer worlds and lose each other.

Support

Support is the ability to sit in the presence of powerful emotions, often negative and painful, without necessarily doing anything.
> **—Pamela Willsey, Program Director,**
> **The Wellness Community**

The daily business of dealing with cancer—the appointments, the arrangements, the mechanics of day-to-day living—often distract our attention away from the more difficult, more basic, and more important aspect of support: just being there. Although support does include attending to daily activities, more importantly it is facing the cancer together and listening to what the other person says, even when what we hear is sad and frightening. The supportive person listens carefully and is attuned to the other person, sits in silence when there is nothing more to say, and doesn't offer empty platitudes. The supportive person accepts the other person's feelings and does nothing that undercuts them. Thus, the most *un*supportive thing a person can say in the cancer world is that there is nothing to worry about: "The CT scan next week is going to be fine. Just relax and don't think about it."

Giving support is more difficult than dealing with day-to-day things because for support to work at all, it must be authentic. Slightly flubbed, it only *looks* like support, but doesn't *feel* like it. The inauthentic gesture feels like bad acting to the person giving it and is hardly convincing for the person receiving it. Authentic support depends on knowing the other person. Unfortunately, however, in giving support, we are guided primarily by our own hearts. We give what *we* would like to be given. This doesn't always work though because our own heart is not always the best guide to our partner's.

A cancer partner told me that it had been hard for her to support her husband in the way he wants to be supported. "He wants to go on with his life and not be a cancer patient, not be worried about his cancer. He doesn't want cancer to be the first thing people think of when they see him." That's hard for her, however, because her husband has a large bandage where his right eye used to be. "I realize that my worrying is not supporting him, but I tend to confuse caring with worrying. Part of caregiving, I think, is maintaining vigilance and watching out that nothing bad ever happens. If he doesn't want to be a cancer patient, I feel as if I need to worry for both of us. When I express all that worry to him, it feels like nagging." What he really wants is to be left alone, so her way of supporting him has been to relieve him of all the responsibilities for housework and childcare. "And now, although I think I am giving him what he wants, I miss him."

Another cancer partner described her early lesson in the meaning of support. She and her husband were driving to his first chemotherapy session; his doctors had recently told them that he could expect to live about three months if he didn't get treatment. They could not be sure that chemotherapy would give him more time. "I remember we were stopped at a traffic light on the way to the hospital, and I started to cry," she said. "'Don't you cry. Don't you dare cry,' he said to me. 'Don't cry?' I sobbed back, 'You have three months to live and you think I have nothing to cry about?'" What he said then made her realize how support has to do with his feelings, not hers. "He told me to think of all the great car trips we had taken over the years. 'Just think of this trip as a journey like those,' he said. He needed the cancer to be a new adventure for him, and he didn't want people around him, especially me, undercutting his confidence by having any doubts about the outcome. I may have felt like crying myself, but that was not supporting him."

"I had to lie to my husband in order to support him," another cancer partner told me. "I knew that I had to support his choice to go for more chemotherapy and that he had every right to do whatever he wanted with his own life. I decided to be as supportive as I could be, but I also knew deep in my heart that the chemotherapy probably would not work. The doctors had already told us as much. I just didn't think I should break my husband's bubble of illusion. If he wanted to believe that chemotherapy would cure him, then I wanted to help him believe. I can only say that my decision to keep up the 'lie' even though I knew better put me in a very painful position. I became estranged emotionally from him at that moment. I felt as if we were living on two different planets. He wanted to continue believing that he would be cured, and I believed that he would not get better. Instead of talking with him about what the future looked like for us and preparing for that future, we had painful and frustrating silence."

These stories are about giving the other person what he or she wants, but they are not about giving that person support. In each of these tales, the cancer partner offered comfort to their partner at the cost of considerable personal sacrifice. One cancer partner misses her husband's participation in the family, another damps down her own feelings in deference to her husband's need to bolster his own confidence, and a third feels growing distance from her husband because, as she said, she had to lie to him about his chances of recovering. All of these things may have been necessary at the time, but they are not support. Support is mutual. It is joining the other person in the fears and sadness, even when we are powerless to do anything about them or to make the other person feel better. It is our acknowledgment to each other that this is where we are, this is really happening.

A feel for this difference between doing something and giving support comes slowly. Guessing what the other person may want us to do is difficult, but we have some obvious clues from the visible world: get something to drink, move a pillow, buy groceries for dinner. And doing something is almost always easier than inaction. Supporting the other person is less a specific act, more fellow feeling than action. We need to feel comfortable ourselves and we need to trust each other before we can give support.

A cancer partner described to me what he called his "bizarre" and "kafka-esque" experience when his wife received her first treatment for multiple myeloma. "We were in an impersonal and sterile hotel room in a strange city far from home. My wife was lying on the bed almost too wiped out by her treatment to sleep. Several times she almost vomited. I sat uncomfortably in the chair in front of the window, afraid that if I lay on the bed, it would disturb her. I watched the sun go down and night come. I sat in the darkness, exhausted, and then I turned on my laptop computer to make some fleeting contact with the outside world. It was my first contact in three days. My world had contracted to the world of the hospital corridors, waiting rooms, our hotel room, and my wife. My only connection to the normal world was by the dim light of the computer screen. The rest of the room was dark. In the middle of this dark void was my wife, lying on her hotel bed unable to get up, unable to eat, unable to sleep, unable to talk. Just lying there. Nothing in my life prepared me for that first time in the hotel room. I wanted to give her support, but it was all too strange."

Distraction Is Not Support

Sometimes we can say the right thing to gently nudge a dark mood toward something more positive. Or we might say something in gentle agreement, joining in the feeling that this really is sad stuff. Trying to change a partner's fear or sadness into something else, however, is presumptuous. Who are we, after all, to tell our partners that there is nothing to be afraid of or that it is pointless to be sad? The only honest thing we can say is that what we are going through *is* frightening and sad.

Nothing is more annoying than hearing the wrong words at a critical time. Watch a parent deal with a child's pain or frustration by trying to distract him or tickle him out of feeling bad. The idea behind this maneuver is to convince the child who has just fallen down that her scraped knee doesn't hurt or that the prohibited candy bar he is fixated on isn't really what he wants. This is a futile and self-defeating strategy. When Trudee was feeling downed by her cancer or the inconveniences and indignities of its treatment, trying to "tickle" her into a different frame of mind would have been foolish, insulting, even cruel. Support takes "the problem" as a given fact of life, and pays more attention to how the person feels. Distraction minimizes that other person.

Yet some partners adopt a strategy of distraction and deception, thinking that this is giving support. One cancer partner I met attempts to support his wife by making her think of other things. "I try to do and say everything I can to keep her from thinking about her cancer," he told me. If his wife says that she is fearful about a particular outcome, he will "try to give her a more positive attitude to take some of the hurt out, some of the fearfulness out of the disease." If she says that she is worried about something new they found on a recent CT scan, he will "try to talk positive because it could be scar tissue. I don't rule out anything unless the doctor tells us definitely that the thing has progressed. Then we have to think about something else to open *that* window a little bit. I'm not lying. I'm just telling her what I think, and I try to build some hope to change her mind. That's how I am. If she ever saw me with a sadder mood, that would indicate that we gave up."

He and I spent a good bit of time together as we made our way through the cancer world. The more we talked about his obsession to keep his wife from thinking about her cancer, the more I realized that he was really talking about himself. *He* was the one who couldn't stand the thought that his wife might be so sick. Whenever she told him she was nervous about a test result, he was the one who couldn't tolerate the anxiety. Under the cover of trying to keep everything positive for her, he was actually hiding from his own despair at the thought of losing her. He built a façade to hide his sadder moods, from *himself*, not just from her.

Another cancer partner, too, told me that his job is to distract his wife from how grave her situation is. "Her tendency is to look at the statistics on breast cancer and say, 'Holy shit, I'm going to die.' She gets her grim news and all the reality part of her cancer from everybody else, so I feel like my role is really to be her cheerleader more than anything else." Despite his best efforts to play the cheerleader, however, his wife still expresses deep worries. She gets up in the middle of the night and walks around the house because her worries keep her awake. Her husband tells her, "From any rational viewpoint, whether you are walking around all night or sleeping or sitting there dwelling on what might happen, you are not going to have any effect on the outcome. It's like when you're in school, and you've taken a test already, and you go back and look at the answers and obsess over what you could have done. You'll see what happens when it happens." He says that although he tells his wife these things to make her feel better, to cheer her up, he can see that his efforts don't work. "There are times when I think she wants something else from me. But I don't really know what it is." He is missing the plain fact that she wants his support, not his cheerleading.

This is where the terrain in the cancer world is particularly treacherous. We are crossing the highest mountains in the central highlands of the cancer world. Remnants of ancient glaciers extend their fingers of ice across the narrow mountain trails that we need to climb as we skirt the summit. If we look up, we can see across the valley to the majestic peaks on the other side. But we don't look up because we are afraid that we will lose our footing on the slippery ice. We have no handholds, and one mis-step can throw one or both of us off the side of the mountain. We are without a guide, negotiating our own worst fears and living with those of the person who is almost our second self.

Trudee described this situation with her own metaphor. She once said to me that she was "constantly walking a tightrope." After a short pause she added, "but so are you." Before we crossed into the cancer world, when one of us was off balance, the other could usually help restore that balance. Inside the cancer world, as Trudee said, "It takes so little, at any moment, to knock one or the other of us off our equilibrium. The real danger comes when the person who is teetering on the tightrope throws the other person off balance as well." Tightrope walkers are doomed to fall when abrupt changes require them to make large adjustments. A single acrobat might be able to make a sudden large change in direction. The only way for an ensemble act to walk from one end of the wire to the other is to make small adjustments while that are not too unsettling to the other people on the wire.

A cancer partner I met complained that his wife "is so engulfed in her cancer" that, although she may recognize how much she is unbalancing other people, she feels entitled not to do anything about it. He told me she says, "I'm sorry if I am causing anybody else disequilibrium, but it's all I can do to keep myself going." She is overwhelmed by the fact that she has cancer; and she believes that the cancer has given her license to act out her fears. "To make matters worse," he said, "she seems to inflict her bad feelings on me as well. As a result, every emotion that I have is amplified, exaggerated. It feels like I'm the one who has to be careful on the tightrope. She is just barely in balance, so I don't want to shake her tightrope. I don't want my own mood swings to knock her off balance because the slightest disturbance on my part can throw her into free fall. I constantly feel off balance because I never know what I'm going to get from her. When I come home, I don't know whether I am going to be greeted by her joy or anger or sullen silence. If it's anger, I have to be able to step away and come back when the time is right, when she doesn't have the force field up. I am so off balance that it is difficult for me to know when to be sad with her and when to lie to her and say that everything is OK, even though I know that everything definitely is not OK."

There are plenty of good reasons for trying to distract the other person and for trying to soften the harsh truth. No one can look awful reality in the face without relief. Denial and distraction are necessities in the cancer world. The man who told his wife not to cry as they were driving to his first chemotherapy was certainly anxious about his future, but he needed to deny those anxieties in order to go through treatment. Yet we also need to respect the truth. We can't let ourselves completely believe the lie. Some realities of the cancer world are inescapable. If our partner is frightened, that is a fact. If she hurts, that is a fact. If the chances of a happy outcome are slim, that is a fact. These facts define the new reality that we call our cancer world, and they recalibrate what we can legitimately hope for.

Distraction also leaves each of the partners alone and separated from each other. The person with the cancer is not feeling supported, and the cancer partner knows that the bravado is only a sham. Once the inauthentic roles are set in this way, each partner is frozen into acting as if he believed the fabricated truth. "My wife's prognosis is not great," a cancer partner told me, "but I have not told her how serious the prognosis really is. I try to get her mind on feeling better and not on the mechanism of the disease." His wife's breast cancer has metastasized to the bones of her neck and rib. She has spots on her liver. Distraction involves this cancer partner in an elaborate deception in which he tries to manage all the information his wife gets. He worries that he and his wife might go to a movie in which one of the characters mentions cancer. He keeps magazine and newspaper articles that might deal with cancer away from her. "I feel rotten about not sharing information with my wife, but I know that she tends to look at things in a negative way. If her numbers bump up a little bit, she becomes tense. When she feels the pain of her arthritis, she is afraid that it is further metastasis to her bone. I don't know if it's a way of looking for attention, but she appears to be very scared all the time. I tell her that the scans have not shown any further development and that she should stop complaining."

But by being so careful to distract his wife, contrary to all her experience, he has alienated himself as well. His wife thinks that he doesn't listen to her because when she tries to tell him of her fears, he denies them. "If she is frightened all the time, I am forced into the role of being the minimizer. I have to be the one who points out that the most recent bone scan did not show anything more advanced. I have to try to keep things down. When do I get a chance to say, 'Oh my God?'"

Unutterable Closeness

Emotional support depends on physical closeness as well. A cancer partner told me that her husband was afraid to be alone in the hospital. "Alone to him was the fear of death. He felt normal and comforted when we were physically close. He felt good when I lay on the bed next to him. It meant to him that I was still his, that I was still his wife despite all that was happening to us. That physical connection between us made him feel whole again."

A man who himself is in the midst of his own long and difficult treatment for multiple myeloma expressed the same feeling from his side of the partnership. "Treatment and the frightening emotions that the treatments provoke come in waves," he said. "Sometimes with repeated treatment like chemo, I can judge the wave sets and ride them the way I used to when I was wind surfing. Other times I just get slammed in the back by the unpredictable wind and the waves of emotion. I go under and don't know if or when I will surface again. I lose touch with what normal is. Just having my wife hold my hand or touch my toe at times like those is a lifeline for me. When I was in the ICU, I knew I was very close to the edge, and for the first time in my life I understood that I didn't want to die alone. Just having my wife hold my hand held my entire life together. Even death would have been OK at that point. Everything I value in my life can be found in the two of us holding hands. It's been a profound lesson about what to hold fast to and what to hold more lightly. It's a hard lesson to learn and hard to express because it doesn't come in words. I can only say that I am grateful to my wife for making that lesson possible."

Another cancer partner described a "very tense time" during her husband's treatment for metastatic prostate cancer. The physicians were certain that none of the conventional treatments would have been any use at all. An unproved experimental treatment was their only hope. For the nine weeks of his treatment, she and her husband were alone together in Washington. She was with him in the hospital all day; she spent her nights at a hotel. "Believe it or not, that was kind of a nice time," she said. "I didn't know if he was going to live or not, but that was a time for just the two of us. All I had to think about was him. Everything else was secondary to our being together."

There is something reassuring about just being together in the cancer world, physically close, in a way very different from erotic closeness. This closeness is as clear and unmistakable as the hug we give a child, or a romp with the dog. When the cancer life succeeds, it does so because this physical clarity is at its heart. It is the foundation on which all the other varieties of closeness are built. Animals may have an analogous feeling when they sit beside each other. The presence of the other is comforting, regardless of what else happens. It is the physical presence that says, "I won't desert you. I am choosing to go through this with you. I will not leave you alone."

"This must be pretty boring for you," Trudee said to me more than once. In truth, I could have done other things, and she knew it. But I didn't want to do those other things. I wanted to be with her. So just sitting there, being with Trudee, to the exclusion of all those other supposedly amusing things, was comforting for me. I don't think she ever caught on to the fact that it was no sacrifice on my part. Quite the contrary.

This way of being with each other does not translate easily into words. The weaknesses of language in carrying the complicated messages we send each other in the cancer world are obvious. If someone doesn't get a joke, for instance, no amount of explaining can make the joke funny. It may become understandable, but that doesn't make it funny. Likewise, the words "I love you" don't mean anything unless they are accompanied by convincing passion. In the same way, the words that pass back and forth between partners in the cancer world barely express the inner reality from which they spring. No wonder, then, that the reassurance of simple physical presence is so prized in the cancer life. We can express a great deal by just sitting quietly together. This is the comfortable sense of sharing a place, appreciating the other person's presence even when it isn't what we might call "enjoyable."

This kind of wordless comfort gives substance to all the other ways we have of giving support—the things we do and the things we say.

The shared silence is what gives substance to taking out the garbage, making a mid-afternoon snack, going to the doctor's appointments . . . the list goes on and on. That is what makes the difference between doing things because they need to be done and doing those same things as an expression of solidarity in the face of terrible threats. One cancer partner's wife needed "never to feel unsupported." His presence was enough to make her feel supported. "I used to sing an Irish song with her," he said, "that had the beautiful line, 'The silence next to you is the softest sound I ever knew.' If she napped or read or dozed, I know she wanted to know that I wasn't far away physically or in spirit."

Wordless physical presence is the only remaining way for another cancer partner to support her husband. "He is afraid a lot of the time because he can no longer understand what's going on. What he needs from me now is my love and support and reassurance and a sense of my being in the experience with him so that he doesn't feel that he's alone. The only way I can do that now is by being close to him physically. He needs a lot of holding, and so do I. So just being close, feeling each other's presence, is very comforting for us both."

For some people, watching a 1930s comedy video might seem like no more than a pleasant waste of time. For Trudee and me, resting from the physical and emotional demands of our cancer world, it was the best use we could make of our time together, given the limitations of her stamina and her need, sometimes, to call it an early night. Watching old movies gave us a chance to sit beside each other quietly, like the old couple we never expected to become. If Trudee fell asleep while Fred Astaire danced up the walls or while Asta scampered off to find the crucial clue, at least we were together.

Other partners, one man told me, would lie on the bed next to each other. He would read the newspaper while she dozed. "Just to be with her was pleasure enough," he said. Another partner told me that he and his wife would "hunker down together" to create times of calm. "We have our little room upstairs where we watch television. We lie down or sit next to each other, and we watch some stupid mystery or British comedy on TV. This is a mindless activity that, maybe in another life, we would not have put up with. But it is very comforting at this point. TV is a good excuse for just sitting there quietly together."

Dealing with cancer drives us back into the trees, where our ancestors probably howled their outrage and gave each other wordless comfort with a touch, a groan, or a sigh. There are also times of tenderness when the two cancer partners offer each other the support of crying out their shared sadness together. Crying, I had thought while we were still barely into the cancer world, would just plunge us deeper into the murk that refused to reduce itself to words. Finding the right words for expressing feelings has always been important to me. But I could not have been more mistaken in discounting the value of crying. As in "songs without words," where the music alone captures the feeling, so can times of crying together touch chords otherwise beyond reach. Crying together is like talking without words.

Trudee and I were watching a television production of Neil Simon's play "Jake's Women." Jake's wife, the love of his life, died suddenly at age 35, and he has limped on with his own life. The play takes place about eight years later. Jake is still visited by thoughts of his wife and the life they had together. We in the audience see her actually visit him in his daily life. The point of the play is his difficult re-integration into the present as a whole person without her. He is stuck in their wonderful past. The miracle of his recovery, as it is called in the play, comes when he is visited by his dead wife, who wants to see how their daughter (now in college) has grown into a young woman. After this visit, his wife is to go back to wherever she has been. He will be free to go on with his own life. He is reluctant but eventually agrees to the visitation because it is his wife's birthday. Mother and daughter are reunited. His wife is about to leave when she suddenly asks for one more favor—presumably her last forever. She asks to kiss her husband. They do. That embrace had such finality that I started to cry hysterically as Trudee and I watched the movie. The play was supposed to be a comedy.

The play touched me precisely in my most painful spot: How can Jake go on with his life and keep the memory of the life he and his wife had enjoyed together? The resolution in the play comes when he lets her go. "How is that a resolution?" I stammered between sobs. Trudee looked at me for a long time, and then tears rolled down her cheeks. She didn't make a sound, she didn't say a word, she didn't even touch me. We sat together facing almost certain disaster, sad beyond endurance. And strengthened somehow by sharing, not trivializing, the deep crosscurrents of what we were feeling.

If crying together can be a social experience, crying separately can be one of the most isolating. Many cancer partners describe how they cry alone, out of reach of each other so that they can hide their feelings from each other. "I cried a lot," one partner told me. "But I always did my crying away from my husband because I knew he wouldn't approve. For him, my tears meant that I thought he wasn't doing well. He wouldn't let me see him cry because for him his tears meant weakness. He didn't want me to think that he was afraid that he wasn't going to make it."

"My husband and I cried together when we first got the news about his diagnosis," a partner told me. "The rush to do his surgery really frightened us and drew us close together. We cried every day. Then, after his surgery, we thought that the cancer threat was behind us. We went right back to our old lives. Then when his cancer came back again, I was very teary, but he was not. I was so saddened by the thought of losing him, all I could do was cry. He was very different the second time. He got into a very solitary mood. He wanted to be left alone to make all the decisions for himself. He was putting on his armor, separating from me, and getting himself in order for whatever decision he would have to make. After that, we never again cried together, and we got further and further apart. I was alone, crying out of my fear and sadness for losing him, and crying out of my loneliness for having already lost him."

An Instinct for Support

Our travel through the cancer world is a tour none of us wants to be on. Perhaps in reaction to that desire to be anywhere but where we are, many cancer partners are reluctant to talk to other travelers. Maybe we see our own fears on their faces. Maybe we think that they themselves are too desperate to be of any help to us. We also may hold so tightly to the other person in our cancer partnership that we cut ourselves off from a great deal of emotional support and practical information that others can give us. This isolation is a serious threat to the cancer partnership because it can be the undoing of the partners themselves.

It is important to remember that talking to other people helps. The willingness to share those bits of information and the stories of our challenges and adventures is what distinguishes the tourist from the traveler. The tourist, like the much-parodied British tourist who just speaks English louder to the uncomprehending non-Brit, is so locked up in himself that he cannot learn anything. The traveler realizes that the real interest is outside himself and is curious about that world.

Although each of us has to invent our own particular solutions, the general ideas behind them may be surprisingly common. I once read a book that was full of hints on every aspect of backpacking, including the advice to cut the margins off your maps. The idea behind that particular piece of advice was that anything you could do to lighten the load and reduce the bulk of what you had to carry was to your advantage. I never did trim my maps, but I did hold on to the idea behind the advice whenever I had to make decisions about what to carry and how to pack it. Trimming the maps seemed too fussy to me, but removing the cardboard cylinder from inside the roll of toilet paper seemed to make good sense. In other words, the line between over-fastidiousness and good sense is a fine one. Each one of us draws that line guided by our personal experience and esthetics.

Talking to a healthcare professional or joining a cancer support group can help partners prepare for our supporting roles by giving us an idea of what to expect. Whether it is tubes or dressings or scars, or whether it's seeing someone we love slightly demented from the medication, or whether it is the sound and smell of vomiting—these things can be very damaging for partners. That damage can have an impact on their ability to be fully present and to support the person with cancer. This can then affect the whole course of the disease for the two people. The cancer partner should think early on about what aspects of the cancer life would be unbearable. The sight of blood, the sound of coughing, helping with the most intimate details of personal hygiene—whatever it is—partners must be able to recognize the limits of how much they can tolerate. And then there is the fear of death. Until we face that fear—and we often can't unless we are in a group of people dealing with death and dying—we are always going to have it. That fear will come up when we least expect it.

The key element in all this support from the outside is the recognition that something has changed profoundly at the very heart of our lives and that, even given this revolution, we will need to establish a new order in our lives. This takes a great deal of deep understanding on the part of everyone. The new normal is so awfully different from the carefree normal we used to have that not everyone can help us make that transition. Without making that transition, however, we are caught in an unending sense of crisis that is even worse.

Talking with other cancer partners at a cancer support group helps us make that transition. We can see how other people make their way in the cancer world. We can get out of ourselves, for the few hours we are in our support group, without getting out of the cancer world entirely. We can laugh (yes, laugh), cry, complain, examine our lives—all with other people who are going through the same things we are. In short, we can help each other understand what we are going through.

Human beings seem to have an innate sense of fairness, at least that is what some philosophers and students of human social evolution think.[1] To be human is to be social. Human beings have been forming social groups ever since they first became recognizable as humans. Around the world, common everyday activities like eating and rearing families are done together in groups rather than in isolation. We defend our friends and loved ones. We don't abandon others who matter to us. We act fairly with strangers. As societies, families, and individuals, we have created many ways for taking care of our own, and we expect that others will take care of us. Such acts of goodness are the price we pay for having moral sentiments. We elicit trust from others "by demonstrating a capacity for altruism," In other words, "human beings have social instincts."

We inherit a moral sense in the same way we inherit the ability to speak. It is part of being human. This biological inheritance shapes such positive ideas as justice, fairness, and altruism and enforces those ideas with the negative feelings of shame and guilt. We simply don't desert wounded mates. People who have studied the evolution of human cooperation maintain that these emotions "are our guarantees of our commitment to each other." Altruism and shame are the innate bonds that hold us together.

Instinct is the operative word here. The pleasant and unpleasant feelings that surround "doing the right thing," according to these observers, are the emotions that guide ethical decisions. We recognize these feelings as the prick of conscience, or in that wonderful

---

1. The following discussion of altruism and the evolution of human cooperation is drawn from Matt Ridley, *The Origins of Virtue: Human Instincts and the Evolution of Cooperation*. New York: Viking Press, 1997. All quotations are from that book.

phrase invented by the medieval writer Michael of Northgate in 1340, "agenbyte of inwit," that is the inborn goad of conscience, understanding, or wisdom when we have our wits about us. We don't reason ourselves into doing the right thing, we just do it because it feels right. "Morality requires an innate capacity for guilt and empathy," a capacity that seems to be part of our human makeup.

Caring

When I was with Trudee during her rounds of chemotherapy, her hospitalizations, just relaxing on our sailboat as it rocked on the mooring, or sitting at home watching an old movie on television, my constant thought was, "I want to fill our every minute together with testimony to how devoted I am to her. I want to compress into what time Trudee and I have left for each other a lifetime of my caring for her and about her." I may have actually told her something like this once or twice, but I wanted beyond the telling that my whole being, whether I was doing something or not, would make all this clear to Trudee.

Support is how we act out that feeling.

The caring is what transmutes the most dreadful aspects of life in the cancer world to something else. This emotional alchemy is how we survive the dangers of our life in that forbidding zone. There is no way to play the role if you don't feel it. The role of the partner is difficult enough without overlays of guilt or reverberations from earlier times. There is no substitute for clarity. The situation demands it. This isn't the only way to play the role. Not every relationship—and not every situation—permits the partner to play the hands-on, loving role. The real point is to understand as clearly as possible what the limits of your love are for the other person. If there are constraints, get other people to do the work as much as possible. Sometimes nurses and other professionals must be brought in. If there are few constraints on your intentions, just the normal ones that limit your energy and patience to something less than infinite, then give it your total being.

"There is something about the physical care, hands-on, intimate, dealing with another person's body, that if done with someone you love, is really walking the walk," said a cancer partner. "You can say 'I love you' all you want, but the doing is what counts." Her husband became very needy in a childlike way because of his brain tumors.

One day, she was away from home for twelve hours, and when she got home, he was literally weeping with wanting to see her. "He reminded me of the way our babies would be crying when I got home at the end of the day. It is very important to me that he know as deeply as he can that he is not alone now." It is very important to her that she know, just as deeply, that he wants her. "Odd," she said, "in the midst of all this fear and doubt that there are these few reassuring certainties."

Trudee had plenty of discomfort during the two and a half years of her illness. I hated to see her nauseated and vomiting after her chemotherapy. I hated to see her depend on her pills to help her through the nausea, to help her sleep, to help her maintain her appetite, to control the pain. It wasn't so much my feeling of impotence, standing idly by while Trudee suffered, that bothered me. It was *watching* her suffer. "Not every pain is cancer," we reminded ourselves. Still, it was hard not to be frightened by the arrival of more or less constant pain. Behind the pain itself was what it might signify.

The odd thing is that when Trudee developed serious pain, it was on her other side. The geography of her body always made the tumor on her left side our true point of reference. "A pain on her right side could mean that it is something else," we told ourselves. "Something else" in our private language was always a reference to those innocent pre-cancer days when eating too much fried food, carrying a heavy piece of furniture awkwardly, or any other innocent misstep might give her a day of discomfort and then go away. Those were the days when nothing mattered. On the other hand, if it wasn't "something else," the frightening implication was that Trudee's new pain was more of the same. "More of the same" is the horror that haunts every person living in the cancer world.

Then came the time when, as Trudee would say, her "evil twin" began to assert itself more vigorously. After months of discomfort, unpleasant fullness, aches, and occasional twinges, Trudee had real pain. This was different from the discomforts that were associated with her treatment. That discomfort—and there was plenty of it—was the price we had to pay for dealing with the disease. This was different.

We made the necessary adjustments. Trudee could only sleep lying on her back. The pressure was too great when she lay on one side or the other, and lying with any pressure at all on her stomach was out of the question. "She will never again sleep in a comfortable position," I acknowledged to myself. The concept began to take shape that some things in our lives would never happen again. This was one of the very few things I never talked about with Trudee.

Through November of 1996, Trudee lived with constant pain. She had difficulty walking up and down the stairs from our bedroom to the living room, so she would make the trip down in the morning and not go upstairs again until bedtime. She sat in her big comfortable chair or she lay on the couch. Trudee's world was becoming more and more constrained as she could physically do less and less. She was having trouble eating. Surgery was scheduled for late November. We believed that the operation would alleviate her eating problem.

Trudee's surgery was a technical success. When the surgeon came to deliver the news, I could have taken bad news alone. When it was good news, I realized how glad I was to have my friend with me. Bad news is to be borne. Good news is social.

The surgery was never expected to be a magic cure. It was our way of buying time. Trudee still had the cancer. Walking, eating, drinking, sitting—everything was painfully difficult for Trudee in her weakened state after the operation. It was hard to know what might be possible for her with a one hundred fifty percent effort and what was clearly impossible with even an infinite effort on Trudee's part. We felt that we could accommodate the difficulties and limits, if we only knew what they were. How to handle the unknown was more difficult.

A week after Trudee's surgery, she could walk only short distances and with great difficulty. What was I to do? I badgered her to walk, but this was forcing her to do something she simply could not do. Walking would presumably get easier in the future. On the other hand, if I didn't get her to walk, that would have other health consequences. No one gave us guidance.

Eating was another problem. Trudee's appetite was marginally improved after her surgery. Still, Trudee didn't relish eating. Should I have forced food on her? Without food (by the time she had the operation, she hadn't really eaten in a month) how could the healing and walking go on?

Then there was the breathing incentive device. After the surgery, Trudee was to blow in the little plastic device that measured the volume of air she was moving in to and out of her lungs. Moving a large volume of air was important if she was to avoid pneumonia. Trudee knew how important using the device was. Still, her use of the breathing device was desultory at best. Should I have hounded her to use it more?

Trudee also had trouble getting the fluids in her body into the right places. During her surgery, the doctors had to pump her full of fluids. As a result, her legs were filled with the excess fluid, as was her abdomen. The doctors gave us various technical explanations for this condition and said that it would go away when she started walking and eating. So those activities that were once so routine, back in that innocent pre-cancer life that we could scarcely remember anymore, took on life-and-death importance after Trudee's surgery.

There was the time after Trudee's surgery when she was already quite sick and needed me to do almost everything for her. With the weight of the fluids she was carrying, her legs were too heavy for her to lift. She couldn't get herself into and out of bed without my lifting her legs for her. The position was an awkward one for me, so it was usually a struggle. I would need to scoop her legs up with my left arm while supporting her back with my right. If I didn't support her, she would fall backward, panicked and in pain. Most of the time we performed this awkward maneuver fairly smoothly. When it went badly, though, it went very badly; and her little cry of pain, indignation, shock, and dismay shot through me like a dart. I felt as much panic as she did. I rushed to get her back to a comfortable position, but often the difficult position was made worse by the way she fell backward. In that instant of recognizing what had happened, feeling out of control, and being unable to set things right again, I got angry at myself, at the cancer, and at Trudee for not trying hard enough.

These things became real points of conflict. As a result, we were both frustrated and unhappy. I was lost. There must be times, I thought, when tough support means you do everything you can to make the partner perform. Was this one of those times? How was a person to know?

After two weeks in the hospital, we drove home from New York to Boston. Getting her into the car and out again was difficult because she was weak and in pain. We did it with good spirits because we believed that both the weakness and the pain were the result of the surgery. Another month of recuperation and she would be just fine we told each other. A little bit more discomfort, considering what it was buying us, was not a big price to pay. So we went on. We both felt a sense of relief that the worst seemed to be behind us.

Then came the time a few weeks later, December 7, 1996, when knockdown, excruciating pain woke Trudee at about six in the morning. We had seen pain before. This was something entirely different. It was agony. Her belly was hard as a rock. She couldn't find any position that would give her even the slightest relief. "Just put a gun to my head," she said, making a gun with her fingers and holding it to her head. "Pow!" She meant it.

If I had had a gun, I might very well have complied with her wishes. I couldn't stand the pain either. Before the cancer, Trudee would say that if she ever got very sick, I should find a way to help her end her life. These were abstract and hypothetical conversations. "If you love me," she would say, "don't let me suffer." Here we were, now, facing the worst of what we had talked about so lightly when it seemed such an impossibility.

When I suggested that we call an ambulance, Trudee demurred, expecting the pain to pass. After ten minutes or so, we both realized that the pain would just not go away. The ambulance came to take Trudee to the emergency room.

Neither one of us had ever been in an ambulance before. By this time, Trudee was barely able to stay conscious. I jumped into the front seat of the ambulance while the crew got her ready for the trip to the emergency department. Trudee and I had driven to that hospital many times. It takes about fifteen minutes. I thought, any second now the driver will climb up into the seat next to me, turn on the flashing lights, start the siren, and tear off for the hospital. To my amazement and horror, everything seemed to be happening in slow motion. They didn't want to leave the curb until they had Trudee's condition somewhat stabilized. That took a painfully long time. No wailing siren, no screech of tires as we sped around corners to the hospital. The short trip from our house to the emergency room took an eternity. Finally, we made it to the hospital.

I stood there in the emergency room, helpless, wishing that Trudee's pain would go away, entreating the doctors and nurses to make it go away. More than frightened: I wanted to cry the cry all over again—that cry of the first discovery when Trudee was diagnosed. I felt as if we had spent our little time of grace and were entering the unthinkable denouement.

With the help of drugs and other interventions, Trudee was given some relief. Easing her pain was a blessing for which we were both grateful. At the same time, however, this experience gave us both a new awareness of what the cancer could do. It sounds foolish to put it this way: We were brought up short by the realization that this cancer can be serious. In the early months and years of our life in the cancer world, the disease was always present but not obtrusive. We could live with it. After this experience of Trudee's pain, there was nothing in our world but the disease. Not even the most aggressive and intelligent application of medicine's vast technology could do much to help.

When we got back home, the hardest thing about Trudee's pain was that I could not stand to see her suffer. Unlike many of the other burdens of the cancer, this was something she had to do entirely alone. About the best I could do was witness her pain. I could do some of the more elementary chores: fix a pillow, help her move in the bed, bring a pain pill, coax her to drink something or eat, help her to and from the commode that was set up in the living room, adjust her oxygen. All of this was helpful, to be sure. None of it touched the central issue of our new lives: Pain.

Pain also drove out almost every other concern. We no longer had those conversations we used to have, either. When we spoke, it was mostly about the practical matters of making Trudee comfortable. Our language of touch was still articulate, but our language of speech was reduced to the brute elements of yes/no, pain/comfort, here?/no, there.

The distribution of responsibility may be a little different in dealing with problems in the cancer world. Trudee and I made all of our big decisions jointly in our pre-cancer life. When we crossed into the cancer world, I found myself forced to operate much more independently within our partnership than I had ever done before. I was authorized, by Trudee and by law, to make life-and-death decisions, for example, if Trudee was no longer able. That was a big one. In smaller ways, too, to continue the example of eating, I was forced to just present foods to Trudee without asking her whether she would like them. Sometimes she just rejected them. I could accept that. Other times, however, she said, "Oh, I never thought of eating that until I saw it in front of me." My biggest triumph was ice-cold apple sliced paper thin.

Only the real possibility of death seemed a new problem. "We cancer people are waiting to get on the bus," Trudee would say. "When you get on the bus, then it's all over." But, of course, we are all walking toward one bus stop or another. Do what we might, eventually some bus will stop for all of us. Every loving partnership is destined to dissolve with one of the partners broken-hearted, with or without cancer. The difference is that the bus stop was a hypothetical in that innocent life. The bus stop is the central feature of the town square in the cancer world.

"Time," wrote Henry David Thoreau, "is the stream I go a-fishing in." Time washes past us and, as Thoreau might have said, it makes no sense to waste your precious energy trying to buck the current and swim upstream. As the two partners blunder about in the sometimes fearsome cancer world, those privileged times of familiar ease are like postcards from home.

I have been a traveler in the cancer world for several years and have come back, much changed by my travels. Trudee and I explored the cancer world together, supporting each other along the way. We struggled to get from one place to another without the benefit of maps. We were lost much of the time. We battled the weather, which can be oppressive one moment and stinging the next. We discovered places of great horror, but their emotional force is weakened in the recounting, the way re-telling a nightmare is never the same as dreaming it. And, to our surprise, we also stumbled upon places of unutterable peace and joy. We found quiet streams deep in the woods of the cancer world, where the yellow beech leaves fell like rain on the slow water in the late-afternoon sun. We found each other.

Still Center of the Cancer World

And central peace, subsisting at the heart
Of endless agitation.
—*William Wordsworth*, The Excursion

rudee's memorial service was in January 1997. She and I compressed the remainder of our lifetime together into the period between her diagnosis in July 1994 and her death.

Every day of the cancer life that Trudee and I lived together heightened our awareness of the loss that was to come. Our knowledge came to us without the buffers that people on the innocent side of the cancer border ordinarily find consoling. As we joined the throng of displaced persons in the cancer world, we couldn't tell ourselves that "things will work out." Unlike the "civilians" on their side of the border who think of dissolution—if they think of it at all—as a distant hypothetical, we could see our dissolution happening, if not tomorrow then certainly before too long.

Yet Trudee and I lived day after day without excluding each other from the cancer worlds each of us had partly created and partly learned to inhabit. I wonder now how we could find the strength and agility to travel through that world with any dignity and grace at all. That we did it with any measure of success at all remains a mystery for me to solve without Trudee's help, now that the cancer world we both endured and created exists for me alone. The meaning of Trudee's travail in the cancer world is now lost forever. The meaning of my own is that I have been altered by the time she and I spent together there.

A character in the Graham Greene novel *The End of the Affair* muses on such an impact of his lover's death, saying: "A week ago I had only to say to her 'Do you remember that first time together and how I hadn't got a shilling for the meter?' and the scene would be there for both of us. Now it was there for me only. She had lost all our memories forever, and it was as though by dying she had robbed me of part of myself. I was losing my individuality. It was the first stage of my own death. . . ."

Many years ago, a group of investigators who were trying to teach chimpanzees to use sign language debated whether to teach a sign for "death" to a distraught mother whose baby chimp had died and had been removed from the cage. They decided not to because, although they probably could have taught the chimp the meaning of such a sign for "not-alive" or "completely-gone," they would not have been able to teach her all the mitigating signs that we humans have to help us contend with death. The chimp would have been taught nothing but the naked concept of separation forever. We are a little better off than the chimp, for we recognize the human desire to extract meaning from such suffering.

Whatever vocabulary we use for capturing that meaning—the systems of philosophy or religion, or intensely personal and private idioms of thought and feeling—living together with fear and suffering and the loss of a person we hold dear proposes *the* human dilemma. Someplace in the recollection of how Trudee and I negotiated our way through the cancer world for those two and a half years has softened my sense of loss. That recollection and pride in having participated with Trudee in her living through such a difficult time and dying as well as she lived, has left a residue with me of something lasting that, for want of a better word, I'll call the *meaning* of what we went through.

The poet W. H. Auden, in his *Musée des Beaux Arts*, captured a truth about how human suffering occurs casually, when "everything turns away/Quite leisurely from the disaster," how it happens when "someone else is eating or opening a window or just walking dully along," how "dogs go on with their doggy life and the torturer's horse/Scratches its innocent behind on a tree." And all the while, some "dreadful martyrdom" is taking place. Cancer partners cannot turn away. We are compelled to witness suffering by virtue of our loving relationship. We are forced to enter into it. We form close loving relationships even though we know that the more we love the other person, the greater the grief at the loss will be.

Trudee was my constant companion and daily concern throughout her illness. Trudee and her cancer gave me the most intense times of pain I have ever known, some of our most delicious moments of funny relief, and flashes of extraordinarily rewarding joy. The cancer was also the substrate of our greatest terrors, gnawing fears, uncertainties, and grief. Caring for her illuminated my life with meaning and gave value to almost everything I did. That caring—hers and mine—resolved the dreadful paradox of that time. We were both investing more and more in what seemed to be a losing proposition, and yet we were also happy. We lived to find comfort in each other. As Trudee got sicker during the last months of her life, she and I intensified the bonds that held us together. The tightening physical constraints that cancer put on our lives redoubled the emotional ties.

The intensity of the feeling Trudee and I had for each other during our very last days in the cancer world has eased somewhat the pain of losing her. As for the rest of the furniture of the cancer world—all the things we could not influence and which eventually did Trudee in— the best I can say is that we had no choice. They weren't our responsibility. The cancer was nothing more than a stupid, blind, mindless accident that happened to us. The cancer itself was devoid of significance. On the other hand, our test as travelers in the cancer world was to create something of value out of that brute fact in our lives.

Just as I had to learn to help Trudee live through the rigors of her disease and its treatment, so I had to learn to help her die. Our lives took on new balance points as we moved from doing what we could for life to striving to ease its end. Although this was neither simple nor easy, it came to feel like the natural next step of what we had been doing. A sad but expected step. Death had been our familiar from the beginning, although we didn't always recognize it. Those last pieces of baggage we continued to lug with us from the other side of the cancer border obscured our view. But as we penetrated to the heart of our cancer world, we saw death differently.

* * * * *

There came a time in the spring of 1996 when our life was beginning to feel different. Trudee and I had always maintained an agnostic position about her future. We could not deny that eventually her disease would have its way, but neither the doctors nor we ourselves could predict when that would happen. Although we could see that things were changing, we could hold the belief that our future was unknowable and avoid the chilling conclusion that the catastrophe was almost upon us. However, as spring approached, holding on to that optimistic who-knows attitude became more difficult. We went through a couple of shocks that forced us to relinquish our optimistic agnosticism.

The first shock was an arbitrary decision on the part of the sponsors of an experimental treatment program to bar Trudee from their study. Her general health was good at that point, and her physicians felt that she was a perfect candidate for the experimental treatment. All that stood between Trudee and this possibly beneficial treatment was an administrative decision on the part of the sponsors to admit her to the study. We were thrown into utter confusion when the committee rejected her for reasons that had nothing to do with her health. Earlier trials of the treatment had had tragic results: a few people had died inexplicably. When the sponsors of the trial revised the treatment protocol and designed a second study, they stipulated that patients who had already gone through more than two kinds of chemotherapy would be ineligible for the experimental treatment. This stipulation disqualified Trudee. She had had that early chemotherapy cocktail known as high-dose ICE, that disastrous first attempt to slap the tumors back, before she underwent several courses of a more conventional treatment. Our hopes were dashed on a technicality.

The hardest part of being rejected was that it seemed so arbitrary. If the doctors had said that Trudee's condition had gotten so much worse that the discomforts and risks of the new treatment were no longer worth her effort, that she should enjoy her final weeks or months in relative comfort, etc., etc., we would have been devastated, but we could have understood the reason for keeping her from the treatment. But we were not ready to handle this decision. It was a committee that barred the way. In one of Trudee's most heart-wrenching comments, she said to me, "I will not beg them for my life."

This was something new to us. Our period of "watchful waiting," as the doctors call it, was the worst time we had gone through until then. The watchfulness was corrosive because what we were waiting for were signs of the disaster to come. We crawled back into the bunker we had fled to when we first learned of Trudee's leiomyosarcoma to await the onslaught of the implacable enemy. There was nothing to do but wait.

The second shock came during this time of waiting. Some of the predictable signs of Trudee's worsening condition began to appear. At the time, Trudee's "evil twin," the retroperitoneal tumor in the back of the space that is filled with abdominal organs, was pushing hard against her left kidney and had just about killed it. Another part of the tumor was draped over a major blood vessel, and the pressure could restrict blood flow to her intestines. If that happened, she would have serious pain for the first time. Another part of the "evil twin" was pushing against the outlet from Trudee's stomach so that it was becoming difficult for her to eat. Eventually nothing would be able to pass out of her stomach. There were also tumors throughout her liver.

The idea of surgery was floated, even though surgery is rarely an option for her kind of advanced leiomyosarcoma. In our case, anything was better than our life in stasis, waiting and watching for signs of the end. Hope prevailed, but perched on the other side of the balance was dread. "I would rather die on the table," Trudee said, "than go on like this. At least I'll be out of it, and I won't know what's happening."

We were told that the operation would take between four and eight hours, depending on how things went. The risk was substantial, her recovery uncertain. But whenever Trudee and I talked about the upcoming surgery, we felt that the very fact that they were willing to go on with such a complicated and risky operation was a vote of confidence in her ability to tolerate the surgery, to recover, and to have a life afterwards. The fact that the medical team and the surgeon were proposing a direct attack on the cancer affirmed, we thought, their sense that she had a future. And if she had a future, then I had one, too.

We also developed our own understanding of what the surgery would accomplish. "If the surgery can remove the "evil twin," we told each other, "it will reset the clock." The immediate eating problems and the longer-range threat to that large blood vessel would be eliminated. "Then we would just have to concentrate on the tumors in the liver. Difficult, but possible."

Everything was set for Trudee's surgery early on a Wednesday morning.

Then, at six o'clock Tuesday evening, just a night's sleep away from the day of Trudee's surgery, the surgeon telephoned us at home to say that he had looked at the most recent MRI and had decided to cancel the surgery. Trudee was on one phone, I was on another while the surgeon explained that the large mass was larger than he had bargained for. This mass was pushing against the superior mesenteric artery that ran through her liver, but he was encouraged to think that he might be able to peel the tumor off the artery. It would be a long and arduous operation, and he wouldn't know until he started whether he would be able to remove the tumor. The problem was that he was afraid Trudee's liver would not be able to withstand the shock of such a long and complicated surgery.

We had known all along that Trudee had nodules in her liver. The CT scan showed that something less than half her liver was affected. According to the surgeon, the MRI now showed that eighty-five percent of her liver was affected. We were overwhelmed by that information. Her liver was very sick and could fail during the operation. She would lose a great deal of blood, and she might no longer be able to make enough of the clotting factors she would need to stop further bleeding. In that event, the prospect was a month or more in intensive care after the operation and still an uncertain future. The surgeon said he felt terrible telling us this at the last minute, but he was firm in his decision. He would not do the operation.

Trudee and I sat beside each other in silence for a long time after we hung up the telephones. We were boxed in, trapped by the implacable growth of the tumors, the natural limitations of what Trudee's body could withstand, and the mechanical limitations of what surgeons can do with their two hands. Our world collapsed to a small circle: just the two of us holding each other. We held each other and we sobbed. Helplessness finally taught us hopelessness.

After several desperate days, Trudee looked up at me and said, "This is getting boring. Let's get on with it." In February 1996, she started another round of chemotherapy, this time as an outpatient, several hours at the Dana-Farber Cancer Institute getting the treatment and then home for the night. This continued for three days. Trudee slept away whole days without eating or drinking. The question hung in the air, more hers than mine, of whether this was worth all the effort.

Summer came, another "chemotherapy holiday." Trudee recovered some of her strength. Again we were standing still as time washed past. We were waiting.

Trudee started to get quite sick in September. She did not want to eat. She would force a small sip of something only because she knew that she needed to. By the middle of the month, she was developing a gastric obstruction. The tumor was not invading anything, but its sheer bulk was now seriously compressing the outlet from her stomach. It was also now pushing outward against the thin sheet of abdominal muscles and causing her considerable pain. The swelling of the "evil twin" was obvious. Trudee could only sleep on her back. She started wearing maternity pants for the comfort the elastic panel would give her. At this point, surgery was the only option, but now even riskier than before. The alternative was to sit still and let the process overwhelm us.

We went to New York for the surgery.

We checked into a sumptuous Fifth Avenue hotel, where Trudee went through her arduous preparation for surgery on November 21, 1997. From the window of our hotel, I could see the Metropolitan Museum of Art just across the street. Trudee stayed on the bed.

Surgery the next day was a brilliant technical success, but her recovery from the surgery was difficult. Because Trudee's liver was not making an important protein, her blood could not hold on to the water in her body long enough to carry it to her kidneys, where it could be excreted. As a result, fluids leaked out of her blood vessels into her tissues and formed a large pool in her abdomen. The doctors told us that this condition would correct itself in time. Fluids were also leaking out of the blood vessels in her legs, so that they were so swollen she couldn't walk. Nurses wrapped them in elastic bandages to keep pressure, and urged her to walk. The physical exercise would help move the water.

The nurses told us that Trudee would not be discharged from the hospital until she could walk three laps around the corridors outside her room. With me pulling her oxygen tank on a little cart, and Trudee hanging on her walker on wheels, she tried to walk. But her legs were leaden, and she was too weak to make much of an effort. I coaxed her, to no avail. She just couldn't do it. Finally, one of the nurses—thinking that Trudee was being lazy—told me that she was going to force Trudee to walk, and that I should support her efforts no matter what Trudee said. I agreed, and the nurse started yelling at Trudee, accusing her of not trying hard enough.

Throughout our time in the cancer world, I watched while unpleasant things were done to Trudee. Watching the nurse upbraid her for not trying enough was the hardest for me to endure. I wanted to hope that Trudee's walking problem was just one more hurdle for her to get over. I wanted to protect Trudee from what seemed like the bullying of the nurse. But I also wanted to believe that the nurse's harshness was a necessary unpleasantness. I wanted to believe that if the nurse could get Trudee up and walking, Trudee would get better. I knew that if she didn't walk, things would only get worse. I also knew that Trudee was trying with all her might, as she had done all the other times.

Trudee almost managed the three laps, and she earned her discharge. We drove home from New York to Boston December 3, on a Tuesday.

The following Saturday, Trudee was awakened at six in the morning with excruciating pain in her abdomen. After a short (and now it seems foolish) disagreement about whether I should call an ambulance, Trudee was taken by ambulance to the emergency room and was admitted to the ICU for a two-week stay. Fluid was still accumulating in her abdomen, and the pressure gave her unbearable pain.

Trudee came home from the hospital December 23. At home, she was attended by a visiting nurse, a physical therapist, an occupational therapist, a home health aide, by her sister (who had come from out of town to stay with us), and by me. It was no longer just the two of us making our way through the cancer world. As never before, we depended almost completely on the institutions of the cancer world. We were no longer two plucky travelers seeing what that strange other world had to offer. We were now intimately part of that world.

On Friday, January 3, Trudee again needed relief from her pain. We could manage, with great difficulty, to go to the emergency room and return home by car several hours later. The following Monday, January 6, it was the same pain all over again. We both knew we had reached the place we had dreaded so much. Neither Trudee nor I feared it, we just did not want to have reached our destination so soon.

We went back to the hospital that Monday morning. The doctors ministered to Trudee's needs and promptly relieved her pain with a relatively small dose of pain medication and by drawing off more of the fluid that was distending her abdomen. She quickly felt much better.

Trudee's two doctors had been devoted, caring, and supportive from the very beginning. One of them, Steve, rushed to the emergency room to see Trudee. He held her hand for a moment and then, with tears in his eyes, asked me to follow him out into the corridor. "We have two choices," he said. "Well, one choice, really: We could admit Trudee to the ICU, where we could keep her alive for maybe another month. The other choice is hospice care."

"For how long?" I asked.

"It probably won't be more than a few days," he told me.

Trudee and I had discussed "the end" from time to time, but always in the abstract. Now it was concrete. As Steve was talking, I kept thinking, "This is it. This is it. OK, here we are." On top of my deep sadness, I also felt a growing focus and resolve. "We just need to get through this next step."

"I am going across the street to see what the hospice center looks like," I told Trudee. We discussed this option. I knew from what one of the people in my cancer support group had said that the hospice center near the hospital was an excellent service. Still, I wanted to see it for myself and be able to tell Trudee what it was like so that she could take part in the decision. "I'll be back in a few minutes with a report," I told her.

While I was visiting the hospice center (which incidentally was very good), Trudee struck up a conversation with one of the nurses in the emergency room. I remember this nurse as being one of the hard-boiled, no-nonsense nurses. She wasn't exactly rough with Trudee, but she did not coddle her, either. I don't know what they talked about, but when I came back to the emergency room, the plan had changed. Trudee would be admitted to the Dana-Farber Cancer Institute rather than to the inpatient hospice I had been looking at. That somewhat rough nurse would wheel Trudee's bed through the labyrinth of hallways from the emergency room to the Dana-Farber.

Yet, even our ultimate days of life in the cancer world carried their charges of surprise. Just before we set out on this journey, that same nurse gave Trudee a large stuffed teddy bear. She had gone down to the hospital gift shop to buy Trudee this parting gift. We set out, with Trudee clutching the teddy bear, the nurse rolling Trudee's hospital bed, Trudee's sister, and me. Nobody spoke.

With a sense of relief on all sides, Trudee was installed in one of the inpatient rooms at the Dana-Farber. She said it felt like coming home, returning to those rooms where she had had so much of her treatment. Nurses and housekeeping staff who had met Trudee over the years welcomed her back with real affection.

Four of us established ourselves in that little hospital room: Trudee, her brother (who had also come in from out of town), her sister, and me. We tacked the love knot to the bulletin board as we always did when Trudee went into the hospital for treatment. At first we chatted a little, but as Trudee's pain medication took effect, she spoke less and less. She slept on her back, more sitting upright than reclining, because the "evil twin" had grown so large that lying down flat was uncomfortable in any position.

I stayed at the hospital with her twenty-three hours a day for four full days. Trudee was comfortable, thanks to very heavy doses of pain medication. Every day, when I would come back from my shower and change of clothes at home, I would bring a book and the day's newspaper. Every day in Trudee's hospital room, I would think, "Why would I take this precious time to read the newspaper?" Instead, I sat with Trudee, holding her hand, sometimes talking to her, sometimes stroking her face and her back. Most of the day and all of the night, I would sit with her just holding her hand while she slept. Touching her hand like this was a familiar feeling in this otherwise bizarre setting. Sitting at concerts or in the movies, I would often feel Trudee's soft, warm hand creep into mine. We would sit through the performance softly holding each other's hand. I held her hand when she got her chemotherapy. I held her hand as we fell asleep.

Nights, Trudee's brother and sister would leave us alone together.

The nurses brought a cot into the room for me, but the cot was too low for me to reach Trudee's hand. Instead, I found that one of the big reclining chairs they used for administering chemotherapy was higher. With the back of the chair down, if I put my body diagonally across the chair, I could get some sleep and still hold Trudee's hand. Touching her like this was the most important thing in my life those nights.

As I sat there with Trudee, the phrase passed through my mind, like a mantra: "Yea, though I walk through the valley of the shadow of death, I will fear no evil." My repetition started there and went no further. I focused on that phrase and I started to wonder what it means to be in the valley of the *shadow* of death. Death is looming and palpable, I think, and is casting its shadow. The shadow is not real, but the death that is coming is all too real.

As I stroked Trudee's hand, I looked closely at her. In her sleep, expressions flickered across her face, moving her eyebrows or her lips ever so slightly, much as an infant's face makes little movements in sleep. I began to see a wonderful relaxation and innocence in Trudee's face as she slept. I hadn't seen that face in years. She had regained a look of complete openness and trust.

At one point, Trudee climbed up out of the stupor of drugs and disease. She opened her eyes, and they were clear. She hadn't been fully awake for a couple of days. Now suddenly there she was, sick but present. I was beside her. She sat upright and said in a clear voice, "Give me a kiss." I did. "Again." She dropped back into that welcome sleep.

Most of the time, Trudee had her hand just lightly draped over mine. Her fingers, which were beginning to get a little puffy, rested gently in the crook of my own hand. Puffed as they were, her hands resembled those of a very young child.

At one point, I had to go out of Trudee's room to discuss something with the nurse at the nurse's station. I introduced myself and, since Trudee and I used different last names, the nurse asked what our relationship was. "I am her father," I said. Then, for a very long pause, I thought that at one level my answer was correct and then I realized that it wasn't. "Her husband, I mean." That was the night before she died.

* * * * *

The second day, a friend who is a doctor, and that friend's medical colleague, came to explain to me the role I could play, if I wanted to, in helping Trudee to an easier death. "It is completely up to you, but if you want to, there are ways to talk to the nurses," the doctor said. "You can make it clear to them that you do not want your wife to suffer. You can take some control of the process and spare Trudee some of the pain."

"What does that mean?" I asked.

"It means that you tell the nurses whenever you think you see that your wife is struggling, whenever there is any sign of her discomfort, whenever you think the dose of the morphine drip ought to be increased."

"Will this hasten Trudee's dying?" I asked.

"Yes," they replied. I told them I would have to think about it.

I did not tell Trudee's brother and sister about my conversation with the two doctors. Even though I recognized that their wishes should be respected, I wanted the decision to be mine and not to be made by a committee vote. I did not want discussion until I had made up my own mind. I felt that the step from saying to doing was such a small one that just mentioning the possibility would make it happen.

Another day went by. Trudee was sinking under the weight of the disease and the morphine. She slept. Her breathing began to get more labored. Watching her struggle like this was painful for all three of us.

Finally, the decision became obvious to me. I didn't know how I would convince them, if I needed to, but I said to the other two, "You know, there are things we can do to make this easier for Trudee." Their instant reply was, "We wondered when you would say that." Still I waited. Hours went by, Trudee continued to struggle, her brother and sister watched me, waiting.

After several hours, I took a deep breath and reached over to the console next to Trudee's bed to push the nurse call button. "Yes?" came the disembodied voice of the intercom. "Would you please come in here?" I managed to say.

After what seemed an eternity, one of the nurses came into the room. "I think my wife is getting a little more agitated," I said to the nurse. She asked me a few questions about what I meant, and then, "Do you think we should raise the morphine dose?" "Yes," I said, almost choking on the words.

What I didn't realize was that raising the morphine dose would not have an immediate, or even a noticeable, effect. The other thing I didn't realize was that the dose would be raised in tiny increments. Having alerted the nurses to my desire that the morphine dose be raised and raised again, I still had to keep reminding them to raise the dose yet again. They would do what I wanted, but I would need to keep telling them that I thought that Trudee's condition was worsening. I thought the code we established required a one-time decision on my part, and then it would remain in force until the end. But the nurses would do nothing without my calling them.

The end eventually came. In the name of our love, I did for Trudee the hardest thing I have ever done in my life: I helped her make the separation from the cancer world that left me wailing in her little room at Dana-Farber. For almost an hour, I sat alone with her, talking to her about our travels. Then I touched her head and said, "Good-bye, babe."

* * * * *

A young woman Trudee and I once met briefly at the house of friends said to me after Trudee died, "Now you know something that the rest of us have yet to learn." Her comment started me thinking. What have I learned from our experience? The one-sentence answer is that I learned that although we think that living with cancer is a unique and bizarre experience, the cancer world is really not so different from many of the other worlds we live in. The only real difference is that the foreshortened sense of time in the cancer world concentrates all our other senses of the place. Highs are more exciting, lows are deeper. For that reason, it is hard to take life in the cancer world for granted. And we are not accustomed to living such intense lives. But that is really not such a bad thing.

I also learned that the cancer world, like the rest of our experience, is a world partly of our own making. There is a concrete reality to that world, of course. For instance, Trudee was outwardly largely unchanged for a long time. But the inward processes were nonetheless going on without our notice. It was the bits of information gleaned from a medical test, a slight change in the conformations of the mass disclosed by the CT scan or MRI, a different twist put on the notion of having cancer that were enough to plummet our confidence or, on those lucky days, to lift us up. All we had were our own ways of constructing the reality of Trudee's cancer. The big surprise for us was that we could have some control over the reality we constructed.

Our wanderings in the cancer world present us with an opportunity to prepare ourselves for the catastrophe that may always happen. Viktor E. Frankl has written eloquently about his experience of living in concentration camps during World War II in *Man's Search for Meaning*. Living in the cancer world and living in a concentration camp bear strong points of resemblance in some fundamental ways. Of course, there is an important difference between the two *events*. The concentration camps were the expression of human evil, while cancer itself has no value. But the *experience* of living in the cancer world is very much like that of being confined in a camp. Not least of the similarities is the feeling, common among survivors of concentration camps, that their experience separated them from the rest of humanity and rendered their words useless to reconnect them. "No explanations are needed for those who have been inside, and the others will understand neither how we felt nor how we feel now," wrote Frankl.

On reflection, however, Frankl realized that survivors had learned an important truth, and one worth making the effort to express to others. The most significant lesson to be told from the camp experience was the paradox that "the hopelessness of our struggle did not detract from its dignity and its meaning." To go through a hopelessly painful experience with another person without trivializing it into futility, and to maintain each other's sense of humanity is an immense ethical challenge. Life in the cancer world is the test of the great human capacity to go on with dignity even knowing that reprieve is unlikely.

When we first met, Trudee gave me a poster with the picture of a gray man huddled inside a gray house filled with the furniture of a gray life. Through the front door of the house we can see a colorful world outside. The caption of the poster said, "Go where life is." This is the greatest of the human freedoms, and the one freedom that cannot be taken away by anyone or anything. It is the freedom, as Frankl says, "to choose one's attitude in any given set of circumstances, to choose one's own way." Even in a concentration camp, according to Frankl, people could say yes to life.

Explanations may be rendered inadequate, but not the effort to give appropriate words to that experience. We can express our fear, pain, or outrage with a scream that comes from the depths of our being. So can a dog or a baboon. What makes us human is that we can transform that scream of rage or pain into something that is larger than ourselves. For this we need language. Failing this, we fall into the sense of personal emptiness and meaninglessness of life that Frankl called "the existential vacuum."

The opposite of this vacuum is what Frankl called "tragic optimism." Tragic optimism is making the best of this necessarily impossible world by "turning suffering into a human achievement and accomplishment," by "deriving from life's transitoriness an incentive to take responsible action." This is not easy, however, and we struggle to avoid such responsibility.

First, we try evasive maneuvers. Shock and numbness are the first evasions. It is simply too unthinkable to deal with being thrust into worlds like the cancer world or the concentration camp world Frankl described. "It can't be. And if it is possible, it can't really be happening to me. Bad things like this don't happen to good people like us."

A second evasion is what Frankl called the "delusion of reprieve." He wrote: "The condemned man, immediately before his execution, gets the illusion that he might be reprieved at the very last minute. We, too, clung to shreds of hope and believed to the last moment that it would not be so bad."

Another evasion is curiosity. Frankl wrote: "Cold curiosity predominated even in Auschwitz, somehow detaching the mind from its surroundings, which came to be regarded with a kind of objectivity. At that time one cultivated this state of mind as a means of protection. We were anxious to know what would happen next; and what would be the consequence, for example, of our standing in the open air, in the chill of late autumn, stark naked, and still wet from the showers."

The most troublesome disconnection from the truth of the present, Frankl wrote, was a kind of silly optimism in the face of the horrors of the concentration camp. "It was the incorrigible optimists who were the most irritating companions," wrote Frankl.

Hope, curiosity, and denial are all necessary in the survival kit we carry in the cancer world. We all need time off from the intensity of that life. "But," in Frankl's words, "in robbing the present of its reality there lay a certain danger. It became easy to overlook the opportunities to make something positive of camp life, opportunities which really did exist. Regarding our 'provisional existence' as unreal was in itself an important factor in causing the prisoners to lose their hold on life; everything in a way became pointless. Such people forget that often it is just such an exceptionally difficult external situation which gives man the opportunity to grow spiritually beyond himself. Instead of taking the camp's difficulties as a test of their inner strength, they did not take their life seriously and despised it as something of no consequence. . . . Life for such people became meaningless."

Eventually, for some people, it was possible to look squarely at the horror and the uncertainty and the irrationality and the unfairness and find something life-affirming. This would not be denial of the horror, nor silly optimism in which one deludes oneself into thinking that reprieve is on the way. This was a way of looking into the worst of it and still finding an opportunity to live. "In spite of all the enforced physical and mental primitiveness of the life in a concentration camp, it was possible for spiritual life to deepen. Sensitive people who were used to a rich intellectual life may have suffered much pain . . . but the damage to their inner selves was less. They were able to retreat from their terrible surroundings to a life of inner riches and spiritual freedom. Only in this way can one explain the apparent paradox that some prisoners of a less hardy make-up often seemed to survive camp life better than did those of a robust nature."

The most important of those inner resources was the singular human emotion of love. Frankl and his wife were put in different camps; and one day early in his imprisonment he found himself clinging mentally to an image of his wife, "imagining it with an uncanny acuteness." He writes: "For the first time in my life I saw the truth as it is set into song by so many poets, proclaimed as the final wisdom by so many thinkers. The truth—that love is the ultimate and the highest goal to which man can aspire. Then I grasped the meaning of the greatest secret that human poetry and human thought and belief have to impart: The salvation of man is through love and in love. . . . In a position of utter desolation, when man cannot express himself in positive action, when his only achievement may consist in enduring his sufferings in the right way—and honorable way—in such a position man can, through loving contemplation of the image he carried of his beloved, achieve fulfillment."

It is a serious mistake for us to think that cancer puts our life on hold or that cancer is an intrusion into our life. Our life with cancer is our life. It may not be our life forever, and there is no reason to make a full-time profession of cancer, but it is as much a part of our real life as having children or taking vacations, taking out the garbage or fixing the roof. The lesson from all this is to treat it accordingly. How you do the cancer part has a lot to do with how everything goes afterward. Even if the worst fears become realities.

Trudee and I did not exactly welcome this challenge, but we accepted the opportunity to give significance to our wandering through the cancer world. This was no conscious decision, but it was deliberate. We never surrendered our life together to the futility of despair. It was our life. The meaning we found in taking responsibility for positive action amid the horror and the rubble got us through so much together, and that devotion that got me through the final legs of the journey was commitment to our partnership itself. We formed it when we joined our lives. Protecting that partnership and nurturing it became a good in its own right. There is something to be said for this kind of trial by fire. In our case, we did manage sometimes to transmute fears, pains, and frustrations into something positive. We incorporated all that stuff into our partnership and, in a strange way, thrived on it.

Regardless of the frightening and painful times Trudee and I went through together, we never let the cancer or the frustrations come between us. Quite the contrary. Trudee and I acted on the belief that she was alive until the very end, not that she was dying. Our behavior may have looked like denial to some, and perhaps it was. We lived but we also acknowledged the decrements of our life as they passed.

At best, we are a witness to the passage of the person we love through a train of events over which we have no control, ultimately. We do what we can in hopes that we can influence the course of events. In that regard, taking the first step in treatment is a tremendous leap of faith that defines the concept of hope. In a heartening number of cases, this leap of faith is rewarded with a happy outcome. In other cases, unfortunately, given the treatment options currently available, the outcome is not as good as we could have hoped. In either case, however, the outcome is not nearly as important as how you get there, whatever that outcome might be.

Even the bitter end will not erase the value derived together from the experience. For Trudee and me, our mutual involvement continued and intensified toward the end. The end of our adventure was not somehow separate from its beginnings. If we had not been threatened by the cancer, would we have lived with such intensity? Probably not. Would we have accepted every day as an opportunity not to be squandered? I doubt it.

The main struggle in the cancer world is that of finding the quiet centers in a world of change. What people on the other side of the border don't readily understand is the flux of life in the cancer world. The Roman philosopher Marcus Aurelius Antoninus summed up the idea in his *Meditations* almost 2,000 years ago: "The universe is change; our life is what our thoughts make it." Every day is different from the days we knew before. It is often impossible to predict what the days will be like, and they often turn out to be better or worse than we expect. The other kind of change that is so difficult to deal with is that of the anticipated or feared trend. Each day is unique, but in our fears they point to dissolution and death. Marcus Aurelius was right: "Our life is what our thoughts make it."

For me now, looking back over those last few years Trudee and I shared, I hate the outcome, but I also recall with deep appreciation a time when she and I lived our best lives. Our "best" lives weren't our most carefree or productive lives. It wasn't fun, like the sabbatical year we always talked about taking in some exotic land but never got to do. It wasn't outwardly productive, either. Trudee stopped working altogether, and I worked less. These were our "best" years because we lived them with a passionate intensity that endowed even the trivial details of our time together with the aura of significance. We learned how to live meaningful lives in which everything mattered. Fun mattered as much as quiet. Pain mattered as much as pleasure. For moments of relief, we gave much thanks. Our time in the cancer world wasn't reduced to a difficult period for us to get through. It was all we had.

The whole experience of being the cancer partner is full of paradoxes. One of them is how I (or anyone in this situation) could feel so attached, to feel even more strongly in love, with someone I knew was going to go away and cause me a great deal of pain. Some people withdraw from each other, making it even worse. How can we redouble our efforts when, in a strictly logical sense, it is a losing proposition? It is a real paradox. People might put on hold the loving to avoid the great pain that they fear is just around the corner. Bu we must face the paradox of loving and pain. We live this way all the time. We are all going to die. The best relationship is going to end with one of the partners having a broken heart. That is a fact of life. Living with that knowledge, *loving* in the valley of the shadow of death, is the greatest good we can do.

I will miss Trudee, the woman who blindfolded me one birthday and drove me to where she had instructed a sign maker to build a neon sign for me, spelling out the Latin words that had become one of our untranslatable jokes: "Mirabile Dictu."

Acknowledgments

I would not have been able to write this book without the help of many people. I am especially indebted to the cancer partners who graciously gave me time for interviews and other conversations at a particularly difficult time in their own lives. Their generosity of spirit in helping me with this book says a lot about how surprisingly cancer can enrich people's lives. I am proud to acknowledge the support of the following cancer partners and people living with cancer: Glenda Alderman, Ellen Baker, Ty Chaney, Jim Dalsimer, Denise Devaney, Alex Fleishman, Deb Glancy, Ralph Green, Manny Hamelburg, Rosemary Hamelburg, Judy Haycock, Steve Kazley, Maggie el-Khoury, Marty Klein, Dean Lavin, Ann Ruth Lipman, Gerri Malter, Susan Merenda, Jim Neely, Evie Park, Rick Park, Warren Rosenberg, Dave Sherr, Ellen Steinbaum, Susan Titus Garnier, Sylvia Winslow, Jeni Yamada-Hanff, and Richard Zeckhauser.

I thank the professionals at the Wellness Community in Newton (Massachusetts) for being there for us when we needed them and for their continuing help as I worked on this book: Pamela S. Willsey, Executive Director of the Wellness Community, and the dedicated facilitators who gave of themselves in interviews and in the cancer support groups they led, Janet M. Cromer, Helen Porter, and Niki Pugach.

Doctors George Demetri and Steven Grossman, at the Dana-Farber Cancer Institute, who helped me write this book by being the compassionate physicians they are and by giving me time from their busy schedules to discuss this book. The psychiatrists at the Dana-Farber Cancer Institute, Deborah Fertig and John Peteet, and the Dana Farber chaplain, Rev. Walter V. Moczynski, were very helpful in helping me clarify some of the psychological and spiritual issues involved in playing the role of the cancer partner.

I owe a great debt of gratitude to Shannon Leuma, not only for being a sensitive reader but an insightful, strong, and tactful editor.

Several friends have played critical roles in getting me started on this project and in clarifying my ideas: Jim Marra, Ed and Jocelyn Mikesh, John and Janet Parenteau, Mildred O. Parenteau, and Peter Salgo. And I thank my friends Ilona Blosfelds, Jim Dalsimer, Mona Gross, Deanne and Steve Morse, Renée and John Randle, Barbara and Peter Rauch, Ernst and Helen Weglein for reading and re-reading various drafts of the manuscript. I thank them for believing that this was something worth doing.

Rebecca, Micaela, and Jeremy—my adult children—were a constant source of strength to me during Trudee's illness. In part, I have written this book for them.

Finally, I wish I did not have to thank my wife, Trudee C. Parenteau, but I do, with all my heart.